DEMOGRAPHICS AND DISEASE

SOURCEBOOK

SECOND EDITION

Health Reference Series

DEMOGRAPHICS AND DISEASE SOURCEBOOK

SECOND EDITION

Basic Consumer Health Information about Demographics and Health, including Social Determinants, Racial and Ethnic Disparities, Genetic Factors, and Socioeconomic Effects on Health Outcomes, as well as Information on Chronic Diseases, Mental Health, and Public Health Concerns across Diverse Populations

Along with Strategies for Improving Health-Care Access and Equity, Understanding Health Research Methodologies, Addressing Cultural Competence in Health Services, and a Directory of Resources for Additional Help and Information

OMNIGRAPHICS
An imprint of Infobase

* * *

OMNIGRAPHICS
An imprint of Infobase
8 The Green
Suite #19225
Dover, DE 19901
www.infobase.com
James Chambers, *Editorial Director*

* * *

ISBN 978-0-7808-2160-6
E-ISBN 978-0-7808-2161-3

Library of Congress Cataloging-in-Publication Data

Names: Chambers, James, editor.

Title: Demographics and disease sourcebook / edited by James Chambers.

Other titles: Ethnicity, race, and disease sourcebook.

Description: Second edition. | Dover, DE: Omnigraphics, an imprint of Infobase, [2025] | Series: Health reference series | Includes index. Summary: "Provides basic consumer health information about demographics and their effects on health, including social determinants, racial and ethnic disparities, genetic factors, chronic diseases, and mental health across diverse populations. Includes an index, a glossary, and a directory of resources for additional information"-- Provided by publisher.

Identifiers: LCCN 2024041641 (print) | LCCN 2024041642 (ebook) | ISBN 9780780821606 (library binding) | ISBN 9780780821613 (eISBN)

Subjects: LCSH: Minorities--Medical care. | Discrimination in medical care. | Minorities–Diseases–Cross-cultural studies.

Classification: LCC RA563.M56 E855 2025 (print) | LCC RA563.M56 (ebook) | DDC 362.1089–dc23/eng/20241023

LC record available at https://lccn.loc.gov/2024041641

LC ebook record available at https://lccn.loc.gov/2024041642

Printed in the United States

Table of Contents

Part 3. Demographic Disparities in Health Status

Part 4. Genetics/Genomics and Demographics

Part 5. Prevalence and Patterns of Common Conditions across Demographic Groups

Part 6. Strategies for Health-Care Improvement and Equity

Preface

ABOUT THIS BOOK

The term "demographics" encompasses various factors such as age, gender, socioeconomic status, and geographical location, which significantly affect health outcomes. Understanding these demographic dynamics is crucial for addressing health disparities and disease prevalence across different populations. For instance, data from the Centers for Disease Control and Prevention (CDC) highlight demographic variations in stroke risk, with some groups having double the risk of others. These differences underscore the need for targeted health interventions to promote health equity and reduce disparities in health outcomes.

Demographics and Disease Sourcebook, Second Edition offers a comprehensive examination of how demographic factors influence health. It explores social determinants of health, racial and ethnic disparities, and the effects of socioeconomic status on health outcomes. The book delves into barriers to health-care access, genetic predispositions, and the role of family medical history in disease risk. It addresses chronic conditions such as cardiovascular disease, cancer, asthma, and mental health disorders, focusing on how demographic variables shape their prevalence. Additionally, the book presents strategies to improve health equity, enhance cultural competence in health care, and expand access to preventive services. The book concludes with a glossary of terms and a directory of resources for further support.

HOW TO USE THIS BOOK

This book is divided into parts and chapters. Parts focus on broad areas of interest. Chapters are devoted to single topics within a part.

Part 1: Understanding Demographics and Disease provides an overview of how demographics—such as age, gender, race, and socioeconomic status—affect health outcomes. It highlights key demographic categories in health research, including youth, aging, and racial inequality, and explores methodologies for analyzing health data, emphasizing cultural and ethical considerations.

Part 2: Social Determinants of Health across Demographic Groups explores the effect of social determinants—such as education, employment, income, and community engagement—on health across various demographic groups. Topics include the role of early childhood development, socioeconomic status, and social cohesion in shaping health outcomes.

Part 3: Demographic Disparities in Health Status examines disparities in health outcomes across diverse demographic groups. It discusses mortality trends, barriers to health-care access, the economic burden of chronic conditions, and the importance of preventive services in addressing these disparities.

Part 4: Genetics/Genomics and Demographics focuses on the relationship between genetics and health outcomes across different demographic groups. It covers topics such as genetic predispositions to disease, the significance of family health history, and the prevalence of genetic conditions within specific populations.

Part 5: Prevalence and Patterns of Common Conditions across Demographic Groups explores how demographic factors contribute to the prevalence of common conditions, including cardiovascular diseases, diabetes, cancer, and mental health disorders. It emphasizes the varying rates of these conditions across racial, ethnic, and socioeconomic groups.

Part 6: Strategies for Health-Care Improvement and Equity presents strategies aimed at enhancing health-care access and promoting health equity. It discusses expanding health insurance coverage, improving health literacy, addressing dietary and physical activity challenges, and promoting culturally competent health services.

Part 7: Additional Help and Information includes a glossary of key terms related to demographics and health, along with a directory of organizations and resources that provide information and support regarding health disparities and equity initiatives.

BIBLIOGRAPHIC NOTE

This volume contains documents and excerpts from publications issued by the following U.S. government agencies: Agency for Healthcare Research and Quality (AHRQ); Centers for Disease Control and Prevention (CDC);

Centers for Medicare & Medicaid Services (CMS); Congressional Research Service (CRS); Health Resources and Services Administration (HRSA); MedlinePlus; National Cancer Institute (NCI); National Heart, Lung, and Blood Institute (NHLBI); National Human Genome Research Institute (NHGRI); National Institute for Occupational Safety and Health (NIOSH); National Institute of Allergy and Infectious Diseases (NIAID); National Institute of Environmental Health Sciences (NIEHS); National Institute of Mental Health (NIMH); National Institute on Aging (NIA); National Institute on Minority Health and Health Disparities (NIMHD); National Institutes of Health (NIH); National Prevention Information Network (NPIN); Occupational Safety and Health Administration (OSHA); Office of Disease Prevention and Health Promotion (ODPHP); Office of Minority Health (OMH); Office of Research on Women's Health (ORWH); Office of the Assistant Secretary for Planning and Evaluation (ASPE); U.S. Census Bureau; U.S. Department of Education (ED); U.S. Department of Health and Human Services (HHS); U.S. Department of the Treasury; U.S. Environmental Protection Agency (EPA); U.S. Equal Employment Opportunity Commission (EEOC); U.S. Food and Drug Administration (FDA); and U.S. Government Accountability Office (GAO).

ABOUT THE *HEALTH REFERENCE SERIES*

The *Health Reference Series* is designed to provide basic medical information for patients, families, caregivers, and the general public. Each volume provides comprehensive coverage on a particular topic. This is especially important for people who may be dealing with a newly diagnosed disease or a chronic disorder in themselves or in a family member. People looking for preventive guidance, information about disease warning signs, medical statistics, and risk factors for health problems will also find answers to their questions in the *Health Reference Series*. The *Series*, however, is not intended to serve as a tool for diagnosing illness, in prescribing treatments, or as a substitute for the physician-patient relationship. All people concerned about medical symptoms or the possibility of disease are encouraged to seek professional care from an appropriate health-care provider.

A NOTE ABOUT SPELLING AND STYLE

Health Reference Series editors use *Stedman's Medical Dictionary* as an authority for questions related to the spelling of medical terms and

The Chicago Manual of Style for questions related to grammatical structures, punctuation, and other editorial concerns. Consistent adherence is not always possible, however, because the individual volumes within the *Series* include many documents from a wide variety of different producers, and the editor's primary goal is to present material from each source as accurately as is possible. This sometimes means that information in different chapters or sections may follow other guidelines and alternate spelling authorities. For example, occasionally a copyright holder may require that eponymous terms be shown in possessive forms (Crohn's disease vs. Crohn disease) or that British spelling norms be retained (leukaemia vs. leukemia).

HEALTH REFERENCE SERIES UPDATE POLICY

The inaugural book in the *Health Reference Series* was the first edition of *Cancer Sourcebook* published in 1989. Since then, the *Series* has been enthusiastically received by librarians and in the medical community. In order to maintain the standard of providing high-quality health information for the layperson, the editorial staff felt it was necessary to implement a policy of updating volumes when warranted.

Medical researchers have been making tremendous strides, and it is the purpose of the *Health Reference Series* to stay current with the most recent advances. Each decision to update a volume is made on an individual basis. Some of the considerations include how much new information is available and the feedback we receive from people who use the books. If there is a topic you would like to see added to the update list, or an area of medical concern you feel has not been adequately addressed, please write to: custserv@infobaselearning.com.

Part 1 | Understanding Demographics and Disease

Chapter 1 | Demographic Turning Points in the United States

The year 2030 marks a demographic turning point for the United States. Beginning that year, all baby boomers will be older than 65, and within the decade, older adults (65 years and older) are projected to outnumber children (under 18 years) for the first time in U.S. history. As the population ages, the United States will experience another demographic milestone. By 2030, immigration is projected to become the primary driver of population growth: more people are expected to be added to the population through net international migration than from natural increase. This shift to net international immigration as the primary driver of population growth results from falling fertility rates and the rising number of deaths in an aging population, rather than a projected increase in international migration. The rapid aging of the population between 2020 and 2040 will have a substantial demographic effect on the country.

Despite slowing growth, the U.S. population is still projected to grow. This continued growth sets the United States apart from some other developed countries, whose populations are expected to barely increase or contract over the next few decades. By the next census, 332.6 million people are projected to be living in the United States. By 2058, the U.S. population is expected to cross the 400-million threshold, with a projected population of 401.3 million people. By that time, the United States will be an older, more racially and ethnically pluralistic society. Non-Hispanic whites are projected to remain the single largest racial or ethnic group throughout the next 40 years. However, beginning in 2045, they are no longer projected to make up the majority of the U.S. population. If the assumptions underlying these projections hold, then the U.S. population is expected to experience several demographic milestones by 2060, as it grows slowly, ages considerably, and becomes more racially and ethnically pluralistic.

HOW DO POPULATIONS GROW?

There are three demographic reasons why populations change: people are born, they die, and they move into or out of a country. Together, the number of births, deaths, and net international migrants make up the total population change over a period of time. Births add to the population, while deaths reduce it. The combination of these two components is called "natural increase" (or sometimes natural decrease when deaths exceed births, leading to a population shrinkage). Migration, the third component, can either add to or subtract from a population, depending on whether more people come into the country than leave it.

Between 2017 and 2060, the U.S. population is projected to grow by 79.0 million people. Where do these people come from? Over that period, it is projected that a total of 181.6 million births will occur, which is more than four times the net international migration. However, these births are offset by a projected 149.1 million deaths, resulting in a natural increase of 32.5 million people. Adding this natural increase to the 46.4 million people from net international migration, the total growth is projected to be 79.0 million over the period from 2017 to 2060.

It is projected that fertility and mortality rates will differ for foreign-born residents, who tend to have higher fertility rates and lower mortality rates than those born in the United States. Historically, foreign-born women have had slightly more children than native-born women (2.2 births compared with 1.9 births on average). Furthermore, birth rates are highest among foreign-born women who are not U.S. citizens (78 births per 1,000 women), followed by naturalized citizens (53 births per 1,000 women). Native women have lower birth rates in comparison (51 births per 1,000 women). Between 2017 and 2060, it is projected that 80.7 percent of all births will be to native mothers, while 19.3 percent will be to foreign-born mothers. Additionally, it is projected that 84.8 percent of all deaths during this period will be among native residents, while 15.2 percent will be among foreign-born residents. The foreign-born typically have lower mortality rates and longer life expectancies than native-born individuals, factors that influence the projected size and demographic composition of the population.

GROWING RACIAL AND ETHNIC PLURALISM

As the population ages and grows more slowly in the coming decades, the United States is projected to continue becoming a more racially and ethnically pluralistic society. This is not a new pattern. In 1900, roughly one in eight people in the United States were of a race other than white. That figure began to rise in 1970. By 1990, nearly one in five people were of a race other than white, and over the next decade, that proportion continued to rise to one in four people. In the coming decades, the racial composition of the population is projected to change even further, with one in three Americans—32 percent of the population—projected to be of a race other than white by 2060.

The fastest-growing racial or ethnic group in the United States is people who identify as Two or More Races, who are projected to grow by approximately 200 percent by 2060. The next fastest-growing group is the Asian population, which is projected to double, followed by Hispanics, whose population will nearly double within the next four decades. In contrast, the only group projected to shrink is the non-Hispanic white population. Between 2016 and 2060, the non-Hispanic white population is expected to contract by about 19 million people, from 198 to 179 million, even as the total U.S. population grows. This decline is driven largely by falling birth rates and a rising number of deaths over time as the non-Hispanic white population ages. The crude birth rate for non-Hispanic whites is projected to be 9 per 1,000 people by 2030, compared with a crude death rate of almost 12 per 1,000 people. In other words, more non-Hispanic whites are projected to die than will be born. Nonetheless, non-Hispanic whites are expected to remain the single largest racial group throughout the next 40 years. Beginning in 2045, however, they are no longer projected to make up the majority of the U.S. population.

A NATION OF IMMIGRANTS

About 44 million people in the United States—around one in seven—were born in another country. However, most residents have immigration in their family history. Approximately 36 million Americans can trace their roots to their parents, while 235 million—or about 75 percent of Americans—can look back to their grandparents' generation or earlier. Although it is easy to think of the foreign-born as a single population, they comprise people from diverse countries and backgrounds. Of the 44 million foreign-born living in the United States in 2016, just under one-half were Hispanic, consistent with estimates from the American Community Survey showing that the majority of the foreign-born in the United States came from Latin America and the Caribbean. About one-quarter of the foreign-born population in 2016 was Asian, and a little under one-fifth was non-Hispanic white. These numbers reflect the current total or stock of foreign-born residents in the United States. The largest sending regions of migrants have been changing recently, however. Among those who arrived before 2000, most came from Latin American countries, followed by Asian countries. Since 2010, that trend has reversed, with Asia replacing Latin America as the largest sending region of migrants to the United States.

PROJECTED TRENDS IN POPULATION SIZE AND GROWTH

Over the next four decades, the U.S. population is projected to grow by 79 million people, from about 326 million in 2017 to 404 million by 2060. By 2058, the U.S. population is expected to cross the 400-million threshold. Although the total population is anticipated to gradually increase over time, the pace of growth is slowing. Since 2010, the population has grown by an average of 2.3 million people per year and is projected to continue growing by the same amount until 2030, when the population is expected to reach approximately 355 million. However, that rate is projected to decline to an average of 1.8 million per year in the following decade, between 2030 and 2040. Additionally, it is projected to fall further to an annual rate of about 1.5 million people between 2040 and 2060.[1]

[1] "Demographic Turning Points for the United States: Population Projections for 2020 to 2060," United States Census Bureau, February 2020. Available online. URL: www.census.gov/content/dam/Census/library/publications/2020/demo/p25-1144.pdf. Accessed September 23, 2024.

Chapter 2 | Key Demographic Categories in Health Research

Chapter Contents

Section 2.1 | Health Disparities in Youth

Health disparities among young people are shaped by a variety of complex and interconnected factors. These issues are often influenced by social determinants such as education, economic status, and where they live, all of which influence their health and academic performance.

Health disparities in youth result from multiple factors, including:

- poverty
- environmental threats
- inadequate access to health care
- individual and behavioral factors
- educational inequalities

Despite significant progress in research, practice, and policy, disparities in youth health risk behaviors persist.

Populations can be defined by factors such as:

- race or ethnicity
- gender
- education or income
- disability
- geographic location (e.g., rural or urban)
- sexual orientation

Health disparities are inequitable and are directly related to the historical and current unequal distribution of social, political, economic, and environmental resources.

THE EDUCATION-HEALTH DISPARITIES LINK

Health disparities are related to inequities in education. Dropping out of school is associated with multiple social and health problems. Overall, individuals with less education are more likely to experience a number of health risks, such as obesity, substance abuse, and intentional and unintentional injury, compared with individuals with more education. Higher levels of education are associated with a longer life and an increased likelihood of obtaining or understanding basic health information and services needed to make appropriate health decisions.

At the same time, good health is associated with academic success. Higher levels of protective health behaviors and lower levels of health risk behaviors have been associated with higher academic grades among high school students.

Health risks such as teenage pregnancy, poor dietary choices, inadequate physical activity, physical and emotional abuse, substance abuse, and gang involvement significantly affect how well students perform in school.

Social determinants of health (SDOH) are nonmedical factors that influence health outcomes. They include the conditions in which people are born, grow, work, live, and age. These forces and systems shape daily life, including economic policies and systems, development agendas, social norms, social policies, and political systems. By addressing social determinants of health, we can improve health risks and reduce disparities and inequities.

ACTION STEPS FOR DISPARITIES

The following action steps have been proposed by the Centers for Disease Control and Prevention (CDC) for consideration by education and health agencies to address health and educational disparities among students.

Focus Programmatic Efforts

- Analyze data to identify which groups of youth are at high risk for targeted problems or risk behaviors.
- Target efforts and resources to support policy and programmatic initiatives that address the needs of youth in high-risk groups.
- Support the design and implementation of evidence-based, culturally and linguistically appropriate interventions and programs that focus on youth at high risk.

Raise Awareness

- Learn more about the causes of disparities and about evidence-based strategies for effectively addressing specific issues among specific groups of youth at high risk.

- Educate policymakers, the public, and other agencies and organizations about health and educational disparities, their causes, and evidence-based strategies for effectively addressing specific issues among specific groups of youth at high risk.

Build Partnerships

- Strengthen and sustain partnerships with agencies and organizations serving youth at high risk.
- Participate in broad coalitions that work to address the root causes of health and educational disparities (e.g., poverty, access to health care, discrimination).
- Actively involve youth at high risk in advisory boards or youth councils that plan programs to address health and educational disparities.

Document Impact

- Monitor health outcomes and behaviors among youth at high risk and, if possible, policies and programs that address these outcomes and behaviors.
- Evaluate activities and programs that focus on youth at high risk and use findings to improve programs.
- Document and share broadly the successes, challenges, and lessons learned in reaching youth at high risk.[1]

Section 2.2 | **The Influence of Sex and Gender on Health**

Sex and gender can influence health in important ways. While sex and gender are distinct concepts, their influence is often inextricably linked. Scientific studies that generate the most complete data consider sex and/or gender influences in study design, data collection and analysis, and reporting of findings.

---

[1] "Health Disparities," Centers for Disease Control and Prevention (CDC), May 26, 2023. Available online. URL: www.cdc.gov/healthyyouth/disparities/index.htm. Accessed September 23, 2024.

Sex is a biological classification encoded in our DNA (deoxyribonucleic acid). Males have XY chromosomes, and females have XX chromosomes. Sex determines whether we are male or female. Every cell in the body has a sex—comprising tissues and organs such as skin, brain, heart, and stomach. Each cell is either male or female, depending on whether the person is a man or a woman.

Gender refers to the socially constructed roles, behaviors, expressions, and identities of girls, women, boys, men, and gender-diverse people. It influences how individuals perceive themselves and each other, as well as how they act and interact. Gender is usually conceptualized as binary (girl/woman and boy/man), yet there is considerable diversity in how individuals and groups understand, experience, and express it.

MENTAL HEALTH

Women are twice as likely as men to experience depression, with some women experiencing mood symptoms related to hormonal changes during puberty, pregnancy, and perimenopause. Women are more likely to admit to negative mood states and to seek treatment for mental health issues, in contrast to men.

SMOKING CESSATION

Women have a harder time quitting smoking than men do. Women metabolize nicotine, the addictive ingredient in tobacco, faster than men. Differences in metabolism may help explain why nicotine replacement therapies, such as patches and gum, work better in men than in women. Men appear to be more sensitive to nicotine's pharmacologic effects related to addiction. Although men are more sensitive than women to nicotine's addiction-related effects, women may be more susceptible than men to non-nicotine factors, such as the sensory and social stimuli associated with smoking.

CARDIOVASCULAR RISK

The blood vessels in a woman's heart are smaller in diameter and much more intricately branched than those of a man. These differences offer one explanation for why women's vessels may become blocked in a different pattern than those in men. Women's heart attack symptoms and the patterns seen on heart screening tests can differ, sometimes leading to a wrong diagnosis or, worse, missing the signs of an oncoming heart attack. Women are often the primary caretakers of children, household needs, and aging family members, and they are more likely to delay prevention and treatment for chronic conditions such as heart disease.

OSTEOPOROSIS

Osteoporosis is more common in women because they have less bone tissue than men and experience a rapid phase of bone loss due to hormonal changes at menopause. Osteoporosis in men older than 50 can go undetected and is often undertreated because patients and providers think of osteoporosis as a "woman's disease."

KNEE ARTHRITIS

Women and girls are more likely to injure their knees when playing sports, in part due to their knee and hip anatomy, imbalanced leg muscle strength, and looser tendons and ligaments. Knee injuries, such as anterior cruciate ligament (ACL) tears, dramatically increase a person's risk of developing osteoarthritis later in life. Walking in high-heeled shoes increases stress on the knee joint, placing women at increased risk of developing osteoarthritis.[1]

Section 2.3 | **Health Challenges Specific to Women**

Women face unique health problems related to human immunodeficiency virus/acquired immunodeficiency syndrome (HIV/AIDS), sexually transmitted infections (STIs), and autoimmune disorders, which disproportionately affect female populations. For example,

---

[1] Office of Research on Women's Health (ORWH), "How SEX and GENDER Influence Health and Disease," National Institutes of Health (NIH), December 11, 2016. Available online. URL: https://orwh.od.nih.gov/sites/orwh/files/docs/SexGenderInfographic_11x17_508.pdf. Accessed September 23, 2024.

genital herpes caused by herpes simplex virus 2 is nearly twice as common among women as among men. Similarly, women account for more cases of chlamydia, lupus, and scleroderma than men.

Even diseases that affect men and women in nearly equal numbers may have unique consequences or complications for women. For instance, women with HIV are at a higher risk of severe gynecological problems, such as chlamydia or bacterial vaginosis, compared to non-infected women. Additionally, women risk transmitting some of these diseases to their children during pregnancy or breastfeeding.

HIV/AIDS

Of the approximately 39.9 million people worldwide infected with HIV, more than half are women. In sub-Saharan Africa, women account for a striking 60 percent of HIV cases. The World Health Organization (WHO) reported in 2023, an estimated 0.63 million people died from HIV-related causes and an estimated 1.3 million people acquired HIV (www.who.int/news-room/fact-sheets/detail/hiv-aids). The Centers for Disease Control and Prevention (CDC) reports that women reporting heterosexual contact accounted for 15 percent of estimated new HIV infections (www.cdc.gov/hiv/data-research/facts-stats/index.html).

Biologically, women are more vulnerable than men to HIV infection from heterosexual intercourse due to substantial mucosal exposure to seminal fluids. Women's risk is increased by other factors, such as non-consensual sex, sex without condoms, and the unknown or high-risk behaviors of their partners—all of which, in many parts of the world, are beyond a woman's control.

Once infected with HIV, women can face obstacles in seeking and receiving treatment. Frequently, they have difficulty accessing health care and often lack social support. They may also encounter challenges that impede their ability to adhere to treatment, such as caring for children or other family members affected by HIV/AIDS. Even when women follow through with treatment, studies have shown that they differ from men in how they metabolize drugs, which could result in unexpected responses to antiretroviral therapy and an increase in adverse reactions to the drugs.

Women also suffer gender-specific consequences of HIV, including recurrent vaginal yeast infections, pelvic inflammatory disease (PID), genital ulcer disease, severe herpes infections, abnormalities related to infection with human papillomavirus (HPV), and vulvar and vaginal carcinomas.

SEXUALLY TRANSMITTED DISEASES

Sexually transmitted diseases (STDs), such as HPV, trichomoniasis, genital herpes, and chlamydia, disproportionately affect women and infants globally and can increase the risk of HIV infection. Latest CDC estimates reveal nearly 68 million STIs in the United States, and 26 million new infections (www.cdc.gov/media/releases/2021/p0125-sexualy-transmitted-infection.html).

In addition to being at higher risk than men of transmitting some STDs, women face specific health challenges as a result of contracting an STD. These challenges include infertility, cancer, and chronic conditions such as PID, especially when STDs go untreated. Women also risk passing on infections during pregnancy or breastfeeding.

AUTOIMMUNE DISEASES

Autoimmune diseases are a group of more than 80 chronic and often disabling illnesses that develop when underlying defects in the immune system lead the body to attack its own organs, tissues, and cells. They affect approximately 8 percent of the U.S. population, but nearly 80 percent of those affected are women. Autoimmune diseases are among the leading causes of death for young and middle-aged women.

Multiple sclerosis (MS), which causes varying degrees of neurological impairment, affects about 0.25–0.35 million people in the United States and almost twice as many women as men. Although the cause of MS is unknown, research increasingly suggests that genetics may play a role in determining a person's susceptibility. Some symptoms of MS are treatable, but there is no cure for the disease.

Lupus is a chronic inflammatory autoimmune disease that can affect the joints, skin, kidneys, blood cells, heart, and lungs. It affects approximately 1.5 million people in the United States, 90 percent of whom are women. Lupus is more common in Black, Hispanic, Native American, and Asian women than in white women.

Rheumatoid arthritis (RA), an inflammatory disease that causes pain, swelling, stiffness, and loss of function in the joints, occurs when the immune system attacks the membrane lining the joints. RA affects about 1.3 million people in the United States and approximately twice as many women as men.

Scleroderma leads to the overproduction of collagen in the skin, tissues beneath the skin, blood vessels, and major organs. Excess collagen forms thick connective tissue that can interfere with the function of affected organs. Approximately, 40,000–165,000 people in the United States have scleroderma, with a higher prevalence in women than in men.[1]

Section 2.4 | Health Disparities among LGBTQ Youth

Lesbian, gay, bisexual, transgender, and queer/questioning (LGBTQ) youth are part of every community, come from all walks of life, and are present in every racial, ethnic, socioeconomic, and geographical group. While many LGBTQ youth transition from childhood to adulthood successfully and become healthy and productive adults, others are negatively influenced by various factors. For LGBTQ youth, social stigma regarding their sexual choices or identities can be particularly challenging. Stigma manifests in many forms, such as discrimination, harassment, family disapproval, social rejection, and violence, which increases the risk of certain negative health outcomes.

For example, young gay and bisexual males have disproportionately high rates of HIV, syphilis, and other sexually transmitted diseases (STDs); adolescent lesbian and bisexual females are more likely to have experienced pregnancy than their heterosexual peers; and transgender youth are more likely to have attempted suicide than their cisgender peers.

[1] "Women's Health," National Institute of Allergy and Infectious Diseases (NIAID), July 16, 2024. Available online. URL: www.niaid.nih.gov/research/womens-health. Accessed September 23, 2024.

Many LGBTQ youth thrive during adolescence, but stigma, discrimination, and other factors put them at increased risk for negative health and life outcomes.

SEXUAL MINORITY YOUTH

Sexual minority youth (SMY) refers to youth who identify as lesbian, gay, or bisexual (LGB), who are not sure of their sexual identity, or who have any same-sex partners.

The Centers for Disease Control and Prevention's (CDC) 2017 Youth Risk Behavior Survey data reveal substantial health disparities among an estimated 2.6 million sexual minority students, placing them at increased risk for negative health outcomes, including HIV infection and other STDs. Students who have sexual contact with both sexes are at higher risk than those with only same-sex sexual contact for multiple sexual risk behaviors.

Compared to their heterosexual peers, sexual minority students are more likely to have:

- been bullied at school
  - 33% LGB students
  - 24% unsure
  - 16% heterosexual
  - 36% have same-sex partners
  - 19% have only opposite-sex partners
- been forced to have sex
  - 22% LGB students
  - 13% unsure
  - 5% heterosexual
  - 30% have same-sex partners
  - 10% have only opposite-sex partners
- felt sad or hopeless
  - 63% LGB students
  - 46% unsure
  - 28% heterosexual
  - 64% have same-sex partners
  - 35% have only opposite-sex partners
- seriously considered suicide
  - 48% LGB students

    - 32% unsure
    - 13% heterosexual
    - 45% have same-sex partners
    - 19% have only opposite-sex partners
- used illicit drugs
    - 23% LGB students
    - 27% unsure
    - 12% heterosexual
    - 36% have same-sex partners
    - 19% have only opposite-sex partners
- misused prescription opioids
    - 24% LGB students
    - 18% unsure
    - 13% heterosexual
    - 35% have same-sex partners
    - 20% have only opposite-sex partners

YOUTH RISK BEHAVIOR SURVEILLANCE TRANSGENDER REPORT

In 2017, 10 states (Colorado, Delaware, Hawaii, Massachusetts, Maryland, Maine, Michigan, Rhode Island, Vermont, and Wisconsin) and 9 large urban school districts (Boston, Cleveland, District of Columbia, Detroit, Broward County, Los Angeles, New York City, San Diego, and San Francisco) piloted a question to measure the proportion of high school students who identify as transgender.

Survey data from population-based samples across selected state and urban school districts indicate that an average of 1.8 percent of high school students identify as transgender. Transgender students are more likely than cisgender students to report violence victimization, substance use, and suicide risk. Although they are generally more likely to report sexual risk behaviors, transgender students are also more likely to report being tested for HIV.[1]

---

[1] "Health Disparities among LGBTQ Youth," Centers for Disease Control and Prevention (CDC), December 20, 2019. Available online. URL: www.cdc.gov/healthyyouth/disparities/health-disparities-among-lgbtq-youth.htm. Accessed September 23, 2024.

Section 2.5 | **Health Disparities in Aging**

Health disparities are differences in any health-related factor—such as disease burden, diagnosis, response to treatment, quality of life, health behaviors, and access to care—that exist among population groups. Health disparities are associated with a broad, complex, and interrelated array of factors, and may reflect:

- age
- race
- ethnicity
- socioeconomic status
- disability status
- identity and expression (e.g., gender, racial, ethnic)
- geographic location (e.g., rural or urban environment)
- education
- health care (e.g., access, quality)
- culture (e.g., norms, traditions, collective responses)
- health behaviors (e.g., smoking, violence, substance abuse)
- biological factors (e.g., sex, chronic inflammation, telomere attrition, cellular senescence)

RESEARCH FRAMEWORK ON HEALTH DISPARITIES IN AGING

In 2015, the National Institute on Aging (NIA) developed and adopted "NIA Health Disparities Research Framework" to stimulate the study of environmental, sociocultural, behavioral, and biological factors that influence health disparities related to aging. Many of these factors are broad, complex, and interrelated.

To address the contribution of these factors to health disparities related to aging, the NIA has supported research that found Alzheimer disease to be more prevalent among African Americans and Hispanics than among other ethnic groups in the United States. Other studies have found that lower socioeconomic status is associated with poorer health and reduced lifespan in the United States. Scientists have also observed sex differences in health and longevity. For example, overall, women live longer than men, but are more likely to develop osteoporosis, depressive symptoms, or to report functional limitations as they age. Men, on the other hand, are more likely to develop heart disease, cancer, or diabetes.

Social environmental factors such as residential segregation, discrimination, immigration, social mobility, work, retirement, education, income, and wealth can also seriously affect health and well-being. Economic circumstances can determine whether an individual can afford quality health care and proper nutrition from early life into old age. Individual and family financial resources and health insurance often determine whether an older adult enters an assisted living facility or nursing home or stays at home to be cared for by family members.

FACTORS CONTRIBUTING TO HEALTH DISPARITIES AMONG OLDER ADULTS

Many complex and interacting factors can affect the health and quality of life of older adults. For example:

Environmental factors related to income, education, occupation, retirement, and wealth may seriously affect key determinants of health over the life course and, ultimately, the health and well-being of older adults.

- Social factors, such as individual and structural forms of discrimination and bias, can shape the everyday experience of individuals from minority or vulnerable populations.
- Cultural factors can have a tremendous influence on approaches for managing stress, dietary preferences, attitudes toward physical activity, and other critical health and coping behaviors.
- Behavioral factors and psychological processes represent major pathways by which environmental and social factors affect health. Optimism, pessimism, and a sense of control serve as risk or resilience factors for affecting health, while chronic stress exposure can enhance vulnerability.
- Biological factors influenced by environmental and sociocultural factors—and transduced through

behavioral processes—may alter the course, severity, and acceleration of disease and disability.

Understanding all these factors and their interconnections is essential for developing and implementing effective interventions to address health disparities among various population groups.

STRATEGIES TO PROMOTE ACTIVE LIFE EXPECTANCY

Life expectancy has increased among all population groups; however, notable disparities remain. For example, African-American men have the lowest life expectancy of all racial and gender population groups in the United States. Additionally, more adults are living with one or multiple chronic conditions that may not affect the length of life but can dramatically affect the quality of life, and significant disparities have been observed in this area as well. For example, African Americans suffer disproportionately from hypertension and prostate cancer, while Hispanics experience higher rates of diabetes.

INCREASING INCLUSION IN AGING RESEARCH

The ability to recruit and retain research participants who are representative of the total U.S. population is essential for conducting rigorous health disparities research related to aging. However, specific racial, ethnic, and socioeconomic population groups have been underrepresented in health-related research, including clinical trials and population-based studies.

SUPPORTING RESEARCH ON WOMEN'S HEALTH

Older women outnumber older men in the United States, and the proportion of the population that is female increases with age. In 2014, women accounted for 56 percent of the population ages 65 and older and for 66 percent of the population ages 85 and older. Despite living longer, older women are more likely to report depressive symptoms or limitations in physical function, are more likely to live alone (a potential indicator or risk factor for isolation, lack of caregivers, or lack of support), and live in poverty at disproportionately high rates. American women also lag significantly behind their counterparts in other higher-income nations regarding longevity, and since 1980, the pace of gains in life expectancy among older U.S. women has slowed markedly compared to that in other industrialized countries.[1]

[1] National Institute on Aging (NIA), "Goal F: Understand Health Disparities Related to Aging and Develop Strategies to Improve the Health Status of Older Adults in Diverse Populations," National Institutes of Health (NIH), May 20, 2020. Available online. URL: www.nia.nih.gov/about/aging-strategic-directions-research/goal-health-disparities-adults. Accessed September 23, 2024.

Chapter 3 | **The Broad Effects of Racial Inequality in the United States**

Racial inequality refers to the unequal distribution of resources, power, and economic opportunity across racial groups within a society. In the United States, discussions about racial inequality often center on economic disparities, but this inequality manifests in various forms that collectively affect the well-being of all Americans. This includes disparities in wealth, education, employment, housing, mobility, health, and rates of incarceration.

EARLY DISPARITIES IN EDUCATION

Racial disparities in outcomes predictive of future success appear early in life. In 2010, math skills at kindergarten entry were over half a standard deviation higher for white students than for Black or Hispanic students, with similar disparities in reading skills. These educational gaps persist in higher education; in 2019, 40 percent of white adults had earned a bachelor's degree compared to just 26, 19, and 17 percent of Black, Hispanic, and American Indian or Alaska Native adults, respectively.

ECONOMIC DISPARITIES

Large educational disparities, coupled with racial discrimination in the labor market, lead to pronounced differences in economic security across racial groups. In 2019, the unemployment rate was 6.1 percent for both Black and American Indian or Alaska Native adults, compared to just 3.3 percent for white adults and 2.7 percent for Asian adults. Similarly, the unemployment rate for Hispanic adults was 4.3 percent, compared to 3.5 percent for non-Hispanics.

Moreover, Black and Hispanic adults continue to have considerably lower earnings than their white or Asian counterparts. Median household income in 2020 was roughly $46,000 and $55,500 for Black and Hispanic workers, respectively, compared to $75,000 and $95,000 for white and Asian households. These earnings differences have changed little since 1970 and contribute significantly to the persistence of the racial wealth gap. In 2019, the median white family had $184,000 in family wealth, compared to just $23,000 and $38,000 for the median Black and Hispanic families, respectively.

Racial disparities in educational and economic outcomes not only affect the well-being of racial and ethnic minorities but also inhibit economic growth for the U.S. economy as a whole, affecting the economic security of all Americans. Research indicates that up to 40 percent of growth in the United States. Gross domestic product (GDP) per capita between 1960 and 2010 can be attributed to increases in the shares of women and Black men working in highly skilled occupations, suggesting that addressing racial and gender disparities can enhance economic outcomes for everyone.

HEALTH DISPARITIES

Racial gaps in well-being extend beyond education and economic security. Health disparities also begin early in life and persist throughout the lifespan. Black and Hispanic Americans face higher rates of child abuse, lead exposure, obesity in childhood, and chronic illness in adulthood than white Americans. These groups often experience restricted access to quality health care, an issue exacerbated by recent global health challenges. Compared to non-Hispanic white Americans, Hispanic, non-Hispanic Black, and American Indian or Alaska Native non-Hispanic Americans are 1.8, 1.7, and 2.1 times more likely to die from coronavirus 2019 (COVID-19), respectively.

Furthermore, the inequitable distribution of health care in the United States negatively affects the health of all Americans, including those with access to high-quality services.

POVERTY AND ITS IMPLICATIONS

People of color in the United States are over-represented in neighborhoods with high poverty rates. In 2019, nearly a quarter of American Indians or Alaska Natives, 21 percent of non-Hispanic Black individuals, and 17 percent of Hispanic individuals lived in high-poverty neighborhoods, defined as Census tracts with a poverty rate of 30 percent or higher. In contrast, only 4 and 6 percent of white and Asian or Pacific-Islander individuals lived in high-poverty neighborhoods. High-poverty areas often lack vital resources and amenities, such as quality schools, accessible grocery stores, reliable public transportation, and safe community spaces, which are essential for residents' success.

DATA LIMITATIONS

While reliable measures and data sources exist to define disparities in many outcomes between racial and ethnic groups over the past 40 years, our ability to trace racial inequality back further and examine the country's progress since the end of slavery is limited by the quality and quantity of available data. For example, significant disparities exist within the Asian-American and Pacific-Islander groups that are often obscured in aggregate data, and data on Native communities is usually inadequate for in-depth analyses. Additionally, measuring contemporary differences in wealth is often constrained by data availability.

Addressing racial inequality requires a comprehensive understanding of its multifaceted nature and the systemic barriers that perpetuate it. Collaborative efforts across sectors can help bridge these gaps and promote a more equitable society.[1]

---

[1] "Racial Inequality in the United States," U.S. Department of the Treasury, July 21, 2022. Available online. URL: https://home.treasury.gov/news/featured-stories/racial-inequality-in-the-united-states. Accessed September 23, 2024.

Chapter 4 | Socioeconomic Trends and Health Coverage in the United States

The U.S. Census Bureau announced that real median household income in 2021 was not statistically different from in 2020. The official poverty rate of 11.6 percent was also not statistically different between 2020 and 2021. The Supplemental Poverty Measure (SPM) rate in 2021 was 7.8 percent, a decrease of 1.4 percentage points from 2020. Meanwhile, the percentage of people with health insurance coverage for all or part of 2021 was 91.7 percent (compared to 91.4 percent in 2020). An estimated 8.3 percent of people, or 27.2 million, did not have health insurance at any point during 2021, according to findings from the 2022 Current Population Survey Annual Social and Economic Supplement (CPS ASEC). That is compared with an estimated 8.6 percent of people, or 28.3 million, who did not have health insurance at any point during 2020.

The official poverty rate in 2021 was 11.6 percent, with 37.9 million people in poverty. Neither the rate nor the number in poverty was significantly different from 2020. The SPM rate in 2021 was 7.8 percent, a decrease of 1.4 percentage points from 2020. This is the lowest SPM poverty rate since estimates were first published in 2009 and the third consecutive annual decline.

In 2021, private health insurance coverage continued to be more prevalent than public coverage, at 66.0 and 35.7 percent, respectively. Some people may have more than one coverage type during the calendar year. Of the subtypes of health insurance, employer-based insurance was the most common subtype, covering 54.3 percent of the population for some or all of the calendar year.

INCOME

Real median household income was $70,784 in 2021, not statistically different from the 2020 estimate of $71,186. Median incomes were highest in the West ($79,430) and the Northeast ($77,472), followed by the Midwest ($71,129) and the South ($63,368) in 2021. The difference in 2021 median household incomes for the Northeast and the West was not statistically significant. None of the regions experienced a statistically significant change in median household income between 2020 and 2021. The differences among the 2020–2021 percent changes in median household income for the regions were not statistically significant.

The Gini index is a statistical measure of income inequality ranging from 0.0 to 1.0. It measures the amount that any two incomes differ, on average, relative to mean income. It is an indicator of how far apart or "spread out" incomes are from one another. A value of 0.0 represents perfect equality, and a value of 1.0 indicates total inequality. Based on the money income Gini index, income inequality increased by 1.2 percent between 2020 and 2021 (from 0.488 to 0.494); this represents the first time the Gini index has shown an annual increase since 2011.

RACE AND HISPANIC ORIGIN

Race data refer to people reporting a single race only. Hispanic people can be of any race.

Real median household incomes in 2021 for non-Hispanic white, Black, Asian, and Hispanic populations were not statistically different from 2020. Among the race groups, Asian households had the highest median income ($101,418) in 2021, followed by non-Hispanic white ($77,999) and Hispanic ($57,981) people. Black households had the lowest median income ($48,297). The differences among the 2020–2021 percentage changes in household median income for the race groups were not statistically significant.

EARNINGS

Between 2020 and 2021, the change in the number of total workers was not statistically significant; however, there was an increase of about 11.1 million full-time, year-round workers (from approximately 106.3 million to 117.4 million), suggesting a shift from working part-time or part-year in 2020 to full-time, year-round work in 2021. The real median earnings of all workers (including part-time and full-time workers) increased 4.6 percent (from $43,461 to $45,470) between 2020 and 2021, while median earnings of those who worked full-time, year-round decreased 4.1 percent, from $58,897 in 2020 to $56,473 in 2021. Consistent with the findings for all full-time, year-round workers, median earnings among men ($61,180) and women ($51,226) who worked full-time, year-round decreased by 4.7 and 4.0 percent, respectively, between 2020 and 2021. The differences between the 2020 and 2021 percentage changes in median earnings of full-time, year-round men and women were not statistically significant.

POVERTY

As defined by the Office of Management and Budget's (OMB) Statistical Policy Directive 14 and updated for inflation using the Consumer Price Index, the weighted average poverty threshold for a family of four in 2021 was $27,740. Visit this web page (www.census.gov/data/tables/time-series/demo/income-poverty/historical-poverty-thresholds.html) for the complete set of thresholds that vary by family size and composition.

OFFICIAL POVERTY MEASURE

The official poverty rate in 2021 was 11.6 percent, with 37.9 million people in poverty. Neither the rate nor the number in poverty was significantly different from 2020. Official poverty rates decreased for people under the age of 18 and increased for people 65 years and older but were not statistically different for those aged 18–64. The majority of demographic groups discussed in this report did not experience significant changes in their official poverty rates between 2020 and 2021.

AGE

The SPM child poverty rates fell 46 percent in 2021, from 9.7 percent in 2020 to 5.2 percent in 2021, a 4.5 percentage-point decline. This is the lowest SPM child poverty rate on record. In 2021, SPM child poverty rates fell for non-Hispanic white (2.7%), Black (8.1%), and Hispanic (8.4%) children, which were also their lowest rates on record. SPM rates for Black and Hispanic children were not statistically different. The SPM rates for Asian children in 2021 were not statistically different from 2020. SPM rates decreased for those aged 18–64, while increasing for people aged 65 and older.

HEALTH INSURANCE

The CPS ASEC asks people about coverage during the previous calendar year. People are considered to be insured if they were covered by any type of health insurance for part or all of the previous calendar year. People are considered uninsured if, for the entire year, they were not covered by any type of insurance. Among the findings:

More people were insured in 2021 than in 2020. In 2021, 8.3 percent of people, or 27.2 million, did not have health insurance at any point during the year, representing a 0.4 percentage-point decrease in the uninsured rate and a 1.1 million drop in the number of uninsured from 2020. In 2021, private health insurance coverage continued to be more prevalent than public coverage, at 66.0 and 35.7 percent, respectively. Of the subtypes of health insurance coverage, employer-based insurance was the most common, covering 54.3 percent of the population for some or all of the calendar year. Between 2020 and 2021, public coverage increased by 1.2 percentage points to 35.7 percent, driven by a 0.9 percentage-point increase in Medicaid coverage. The uninsured rate among children under age 19 decreased by 0.6 percentage points to 5.0 percent between 2020 and 2021. During that period, there was a 1.3 percentage-point increase in public coverage of children under age 19. Between 2020 and 2021, public coverage rates increased for all workers aged 15–64. Among full-time, year-round workers, 7.9 percent had public health insurance in 2021, up 1.8 percentage points from 2020, in part due to the changing composition of the labor force through the pandemic and following the 2020 recession.

Among part-time or part-year workers, the percentage with public coverage increased 1.6 percentage points to 22.6 percent during this period, which may be related to policies to address the coronavirus 2019 (COVID-19) public health emergency.

This report highlights significant trends in income, poverty, and health insurance coverage in the United States for 2021. It illustrates the stability of median household income and fluctuations in poverty rates among different demographic groups. The findings indicate ongoing challenges related to health insurance coverage, particularly among specific populations.[1]

[1] "Income, Poverty, and Health Insurance Coverage in the United States: 2021," United States Census Bureau, September 13, 2022. Available online. URL: www.census.gov/newsroom/press-releases/2022/income-poverty-health-insurance-coverage.html. Accessed September 24, 2024.

Chapter 5 | **Health Disparities in Rural Communities**

RURAL PUBLIC HEALTH

Rural public health is the science and practice of preventing disease, prolonging life, and promoting health and well-being in rural communities. It seeks to protect community health and works with rural health-care systems to improve the overall quality of life for every individual.

One in five people in the United States live in rural areas. Several demographic, environmental, economic, and social factors may put rural residents at higher risk of death than those living in urban areas. This is especially true for the top five leading causes of death:

- heart disease
- cancer
- unintentional injury
- chronic lower respiratory disease
- stroke

WHY RURAL RESIDENTS ARE AT GREATER RISK

People who live in rural areas in the United States tend to be older and sicker than their urban counterparts. Rural residents have higher rates of cigarette smoking, high blood pressure (HBP), and obesity. They also experience higher rates of poverty, less access to health care, and are less likely to have health insurance.

Unintentional injury deaths are more common in rural areas than in urban areas, partially due to motor vehicle crashes and opioid overdoses. Understanding the health dangers faced by rural residents is crucial for those living in these areas.

HOW IT AFFECTS LIVES

Drug Overdose in Rural America

Drug overdoses are the leading cause of injury or death in the United States, resulting in approximately 52,000 deaths in 2015. In rural areas, rates of drug overdose deaths are rising and have surpassed those in urban areas.

While rural areas report a lower percentage of people engaging in illicit drug use compared to urban areas, the effects of such use are more pronounced. Among individuals who have used illicit drugs in the past year, the prevalence of drug use disorders is similar in both rural and urban settings.

Most rural overdose deaths occur at home, where rescue efforts may fall to relatives who often have limited knowledge of or access to naloxone and overdose follow-up care.

Suicide in Rural America

Suicide is a leading cause of death in the United States, responsible for over 48,000 deaths in 2021—approximately one suicide every 11 minutes.

In the past two decades, suicide rates have consistently been higher in rural areas than in urban areas. Between 2000 and 2020, suicide rates increased by 46 percent in non-metro areas compared to 27.3 percent in metro areas. Non-Hispanic white individuals have the highest suicide rates in urban areas, while non-Hispanic American Indian and Alaska Native people have the highest rates in rural areas. Moreover, rural residents have 1.5 times the rate of emergency department visits for nonfatal self-harm compared to urban residents.

FACTORS CONTRIBUTING TO HIGHER HEALTH RISKS

The following demographic, environmental, economic, and social factors may contribute to higher mortality risk from public health conditions among rural residents:

- older age and more illness than their urban counterparts

- higher rates of cigarette smoking, HBP, and obesity
- less leisure-time physical activity and lower seat-belt use
- higher rates of poverty
- less access to health care and health insurance

PRIORITIES

The gaps in health in rural America can be addressed and improved. Health-care providers in rural areas can take the following actions:

- Screen patients for HBP and set blood pressure control as an improvement goal.
- Increase cancer prevention and early detection efforts.
- Encourage physical activity and healthy eating to reduce obesity.
- Promote smoking cessation.
- Share resources with families who have children with mental, behavioral, or developmental disorders.
- Promote motor vehicle safety.
- Treat opioid use disorder.

Rural public health initiatives must focus on addressing the unique challenges faced by rural communities to improve health outcomes and reduce disparities.[1]

[1] "About Rural Health," Centers for Disease Control and Prevention (CDC), May 16, 2024. Available online. URL: www.cdc.gov/rural-health/php/about/index.html. Accessed September 25, 2024.

Chapter 6 | The Effects of Climate Change on Health and Well-Being

CLIMATE CHANGE

Changes in the Earth's climate can affect public health, agriculture, water supplies, energy production and use, land use and development, and recreation. The nature and extent of these effects, and whether they will be harmful or beneficial, will vary regionally and over time. Because effects on human health are complex, often indirect, and dependent on multiple societal and environmental factors (including how people respond to these effects), the development of appropriate health-related climate indicators is challenging and still emerging. It is important for health-related climate indicators to be clear, measurable, and timely to better understand the link between climate change and health effects.

Changes in climate affect the average weather conditions to which we are accustomed. These changes can result in multiple threats to human health and welfare. Warmer average temperatures will likely lead to hotter days and more frequent and longer heat waves, which could increase the number of heat-related illnesses and deaths. Increases in the frequency or severity of extreme weather events, such as storms, could increase the risk of dangerous flooding, high winds, and other direct threats to people and property. Warmer temperatures could also reduce air quality by increasing the chemical reactions that produce smog and, along with changes in precipitation patterns and extreme events, could enhance the spread of some diseases.

In addition, climate change could require adaptation on larger and faster scales than in the past, presenting challenges to human well-being and the economy. The more extensively and more rapidly the climate changes, the larger the potential effects on society. The extent to which climate change will affect different regions and sectors of society will depend not only on the sensitivity of those systems to climate change but also on their ability to adapt to or cope with climate change. Populations of particular concern include the poor, the elderly, those already in poor health, the disabled, and indigenous populations.[1]

HEALTH EFFECTS OF CLIMATE CHANGE

Among the health effects cited by the 2018 National Climate Assessment are the following:

- Atmospheric warming has the potential to increase ground-level ozone in many regions, which can cause multiple health issues (such as bronchitis, emphysema, and asthma) and worsen lung function.
- Higher summer temperatures are linked to an increased risk of heat-related illnesses and death. Older adults, pregnant women, and children are at particular risk, as are people living in urban areas because of the additional heat associated with urban heat islands.
- Climate change is expected to expose more people to ticks that carry Lyme disease or other bacterial and viral agents, and to mosquitoes that transmit West Nile and other viruses.
- More frequent extreme weather events such as droughts, hurricanes, floods, and wildfires will not only put people's lives at risk but can also worsen underlying medical conditions, increase stress, and lead to adverse mental health effects.

[1] "Climate Change Indicators: Health and Society," U.S. Environmental Protection Agency (EPA), June 27, 2024. Available online. URL: www.epa.gov/climate-indicators/health-society. Accessed September 23, 2024.

- Rising temperatures and extreme weather have the potential to disrupt the availability, safety, and nutritional quality of food.[2]

Heat-Related Deaths

Since 1979, more than 14,000 Americans have died directly from heat-related causes, according to death certificates. The annual death rate is higher when accounting for deaths in which heat was reported as a contributing factor, including the interaction of heat and cardiovascular disease. People aged 65 and older are a particular concern: a growing demographic group that is several times more likely to die from heat-related cardiovascular disease than the general population. Considerable year-to-year variability and certain limitations of the underlying data for this indicator make it difficult to determine whether the United States has experienced long-term trends in the number of deaths classified as "heat-related."

Heat-Related Workplace Deaths

Outdoor workers, particularly those engaging in strenuous physical activity, disproportionately face greater heat-related health threats. From 1992 to 2022, a total of 986 workers across all industry sectors in the United States died from exposure to heat. This represents an average of 34 deaths per year. In the same period, 334 construction workers lost their lives to heat exposure on the job—meaning that the construction sector accounted for about 34 percent of all occupational heat-related deaths.

Heat-Related Illnesses

From 2001 to 2010, about 28,000 heat-related hospitalizations were recorded across 20 states. Annual rates ranged from fewer than one case per 100,000 people in some states to nearly four cases per

[2] "Frequently Asked Questions about Climate Change," U.S. Environmental Protection Agency (EPA), February 12, 2024. Available online. URL: www.epa.gov/climatechange-science/frequently-asked-questions-about-climate-change#health. Accessed September 23, 2024.

100,000 people in others. People aged 65 and older accounted for more heat-related hospitalizations than any other age group from 2001 to 2010, and males were hospitalized for heat-related illnesses more than twice as often as females.

Cold-Related Deaths

Since 1979, more than 19,000 Americans have been reported to have died from exposure to cold temperatures. The annual death rate is higher when accounting for deaths in which cold was reported as a contributing factor. Some winter deaths are due to factors other than exposure to cold conditions (such as the flu). In other cases, even if cold exposure contributes to a death, it may not be reported as "cold-related" on a death certificate. These limitations, as well as year-to-year variability in the data and a change in classification codes in the late 1990s, make it difficult to determine whether the United States has experienced long-term trends in the number of deaths classified as "cold-related."

Heating and Cooling Degree Days

Heating and cooling degree days measure the difference between outdoor temperatures and the temperatures that people find comfortable indoors. As the U.S. climate has warmed in recent years, heating degree days have decreased, and cooling degree days have increased overall, suggesting that Americans need to use less energy for heating and more energy for air conditioning. This pattern stands out the most in the North and West, while much of the Southeast has experienced the opposite results.

Lyme Disease

Lyme disease is a bacterial illness spread by ticks that bite humans. Many factors influence tick habitat and populations, including climate. Nationwide, the rate of reported cases of Lyme disease has nearly doubled since 1991. The number and distribution of reported cases of Lyme disease have increased in the Northeast and upper Midwest over time, where some states now report 50–110 more cases of Lyme disease per 100,000 people than they did in 1991.

West Nile Virus

West Nile virus (WNV) is spread by mosquitoes, whose habitat and populations are influenced by temperature and water availability. The incidence of WNV neuroinvasive disease in the United States has varied widely from year to year and among geographic regions since tracking began in 2002. Variation in disease incidence is affected by climate and many other factors, and no obvious long-term trend can be detected yet through this limited data set.[3]

[3] See footnote [1].

Chapter 7 | **Health Data and Research Methodologies**

Chapter Contents

Section 7.1 | National Health Interview Survey (NHIS)

The National Health Interview Survey (NHIS) has monitored the health of the nation since 1957. NHIS data are collected through personal household interviews. For over 50 years, interviewers from the U.S. Census Bureau have visited American homes to ask about a broad range of health topics. Survey results have been instrumental in providing data to track health status, health-care access, and progress toward achieving national health objectives.

IMPORTANCE OF THE SURVEY

The main objective of the NHIS is to monitor the health of the U.S. population through the collection and analysis of data on a broad range of health topics, such as medical conditions, health insurance, doctor visits, physical activity, and other health behaviors. The National Health Interview Survey data are used to monitor progress toward national health objectives, evaluate health policies and programs, and track changes in health behaviors and health-care use. Government agencies, universities, private health planners, and researchers use the data to identify and address significant health problems. The data are also used to determine how best to utilize available resources to resolve these health issues.

WHAT TO EXPECT IF SELECTED FOR THE SURVEY

A household selected for the National Health Interview Survey will first receive a letter from the director of the National Center for Health Statistics. The letter provides information about the survey and informs the resident(s) that they can expect to be contacted by a Census Bureau interviewer in the near future. The Census Bureau interviewer will conduct the interview at the respondent's convenience. This means that if the respondent works, the interview can be conducted after business hours or on the weekend. If daytime is preferable, that time can also be accommodated. The survey takes an average of about one hour to complete, depending on the size and health of family members. The survey covers a wide range of topics, such as doctor visits, medical conditions, health insurance, physical activity, and injuries. Questions are also included to help better understand the health information provided. For example, inquiries may include race, income, and permission to combine responses with information from other sources, such as medical records. Most people do not experience difficulty with the questions in the NHIS; however, some may find certain questions to be sensitive. Respondents are not obligated to answer any questions they do not wish to address.

SELECTION PROCESS FOR THE SURVEY

The Census Bureau selected addresses across the entire country using scientific methods to ensure representation of all communities. Your household was selected to represent thousands of other households like yours. If participation does not occur, no alternative households can be selected, potentially resulting in underrepresentation in national estimates. These estimates are used by policymakers to determine the needs for health services in the country. By participating, a valuable public service is performed for the family, community, and country.

VERIFICATION OF ADDRESS SELECTION

To verify that your address was selected for this survey, you can contact your Census Bureau Regional Office. They can confirm whether your address was selected for a specific survey.

VERIFICATION OF CENSUS BUREAU EMPLOYEE

All Census Bureau employees identify themselves by name and carry a badge identifying them as U.S. Census Bureau employees. They will also carry a laptop with the Census Bureau logo to conduct the survey. If a call is received and there is a desire to verify the caller's identity as a Census Bureau employee, you can contact one of the regional offices or use the staff search on the website.

IMPORTANCE OF PARTICIPATION IN A HEALTH SURVEY

This survey focuses on the nation's health. It seeks to understand how many people are sick and why they are sick, as well as how many people are healthy and what contributes to their health. Everyone's responses are significant.

PARTICIPATION REQUIREMENT

Participation in the survey is voluntary; however, if a selected individual does not participate, no replacement can be selected, which may lead to the underrepresentation of households similar to theirs in national estimates.

SAFETY OF RESPONSES

Responses collected from surveys conducted by Census Bureau field representatives and contact center staff are encrypted both in transit and at rest on the Census Bureau's servers. These servers are part of a stand-alone network that is not accessible via the Internet and are constantly monitored for any signs of intrusion.

ADDITIONAL QUESTIONS OR ISSUES

For any additional questions about the survey, or to speak with someone at the Census Bureau, individuals can contact the respondent advocate. The respondent advocate can address the concerns of households selected to participate in this survey and share feedback with those managing the survey operations.[1]

Section 7.2 | Demographic Analysis and Post-Enumeration Surveys

COVERAGE MEASUREMENT IN THE U.S. CENSUS

The U.S. Census Bureau has a long history of evaluating population coverage in decennial censuses. Formal evaluations began with the 1940 Census. Almost everything we know about the size of the

[1] "National Health Interview Survey (NHIS)," United States Census Bureau, October 28, 2021. Available online. URL: www.census.gov/programs-surveys/nhis.html. Accessed September 24, 2024.

coverage error, trends in census coverage, and differences among subgroups of the population comes from the Census Bureau's own evaluation programs.

Two principal methods are used to measure coverage in censuses. One method derives coverage estimates from the Post-Enumeration Survey (PES) using dual system estimation. The other method is called "Demographic Analysis" (DA). DA represents a macro-level approach, where population estimates are developed for the census date by aggregating various types of demographic data.

A coverage measurement program is essential for measuring the effectiveness of any census, including the 2020 Census, in terms of data quality. Coverage measures must be produced to determine whether the 2020 goals were met and to establish how future censuses can be improved.

DEMOGRAPHIC ANALYSIS

Demographic Analysis is used to evaluate the quality of the census. It utilizes current and historical vital records, data on international migration, and Medicare records to produce national estimates of the population on April 1 by age, sex, DA race categories, and Hispanic origin. The DA population estimates are independent of the decennial census. The results are used to produce estimates of net coverage error, calculated as the percent difference between the census counts and the DA population estimates:

Net Coverage Error = 100 × [(Census Count – DA Estimate)/ DA Estimate]

Traditionally, the DA estimates have been produced by sex and single year of age for the race categories Black and non-Black. Starting in 2010, the DA program produces estimates by Hispanic origin (Hispanic/Non-Hispanic) for a limited number of ages. New data sources, changes in the racial and ethnic makeup of the nation, and evolving patterns of international migration present both challenges and opportunities for DA.

2020 Demographic Analysis

The experimental state and county DA estimates of population and net coverage error for children aged zero to four were released on April 11, 2024. Net coverage error is calculated as the percent difference between the census count and the DA estimate.

On March 10, 2022, the national DA net coverage error estimates by age and sex for the 2020 Census were released at a news conference. This release included DA net coverage error estimates by sex and:

1. a single year of age
2. five-year age groups and sex
3. the selected age groups used by the PES

A range of net coverage error estimates—low, middle, and high—was released to account for uncertainty in the data and methods used to produce the DA population estimates.

The DA estimates for April 1, 2020, were released at a news conference on December 15, 2020. This release included three official sets of DA estimates for the Black Alone/Non-Black Alone, Black Alone or in Combination/Non-Black Alone or in Combination, and Hispanic/Non-Hispanic populations by single year of age and sex. A range of estimates—low, middle, and high—was produced for each set to account for uncertainty.

POST-ENUMERATION SURVEYS

The purpose of the PES is to measure the accuracy of the census. This survey measures the accuracy of the census by independently surveying a sample of the population.

Since 1980, the U.S. Census Bureau has used PES with dual system estimation to measure coverage in the Decennial Censuses of Population and Housing. This approach involves case-by-case matching of people in an independent survey with people in the census to determine who was missed or counted in error.

2020 Post-Enumeration Surveys

The 2020 PES was designed to support national-level and state-level estimates of census coverage. Its primary goal was to measure coverage errors in the 2020 Census. Fieldwork for the 2020 PES began in January 2020 and ended in February 2022.[1]

[1] "Coverage Measurement," United States Census Bureau, May 19, 2022. Available online. URL: www.census.gov/programs-surveys/decennial-census/about/coverage-measurement.html. Accessed September 25, 2024.

Section 7.3 | National Electronic Health Records Survey (NEHRS)

The National Electronic Health Records Survey (NEHRS) is an annual survey that measures the progress U.S. physicians and their offices have made in adopting electronic health records (EHRs). The survey also monitors health information exchange, including interoperability, and the burden associated with EHRs.

Health information exchange is the sharing of health record information between and among different providers and facilities. Electronic health records systems are considered interoperable when they can share usable information directly from system to system.

The NEHRS began in 2008 as an annual mail supplement to the National Ambulatory Medical Care Survey (NAMCS). In 2010, it expanded to measure EHR adoption rates across all 50 U.S. states and the District of Columbia. In 2012, it became a standalone survey conducted separately from the NAMCS.

The Office of the National Coordinator for Health Information Technology sponsors the NEHRS, which is conducted by the National Center for Health Statistics (NCHS) in collaboration with RTI International, a nonprofit research organization.

DATA COLLECTION

The NEHRS collects data about electronic health record use from office-based physicians practicing in the United States. It does not collect data from physicians employed by the federal government, anesthesiologists, radiologists, or pathologists.

Currently, the NCHS collects NEHRS data through a web survey and paper questionnaire. Previously, it also collected the data by telephone.

DATA AND DOCUMENTATION

The NCHS publishes the NEHRS reports and summary web tables describing the number of physicians who have adopted EHRs and the rate at which they are adopting these systems. In producing these resources, the NEHRS staff prioritize protecting the privacy of providers and practices.

PUBLIC USE AND RESTRICTED DATA FILES

Public use data files (PUFs) are available for download. To ensure the confidentiality of respondents, all potentially identifiable information about providers has been removed from PUFs.

Investigators must submit requests through the Standard Application Process portal to access restricted NEHRS data. Restricted data files are available for a fee through the NCHS Research Data Center (RDC), which provides instructions for preparing and submitting an application to access restricted data.

USE OF DATA

Results from the NEHRS provide data to track the adoption and use of EHR systems. Researchers can use the NEHRS data to produce state and national estimates of adoption, capabilities, and burden.

The NEHRS also monitors physicians' progress toward meeting the policy goals of the Health Information Technology for Economic and Clinical Health (HITECH) Act.

In recent years, survey data have been used to:

- measure the sharing of patient health information
- track participation in the Centers for Medicare and Medicaid Services' promoting interoperability programs
- analyze trends in reports such as *Health, United States* and Healthy People
- advance federal, public, and international research

PARTICIPATION INSTRUCTIONS

To access the 2024 NEHRS survey, visit https://providerehr.cdc.gov if selected to participate.

If a physician receives the survey, they can either answer the questions themselves or identify a knowledgeable member of the office staff to complete it.

Completing the NEHRS questionnaire should take about 20 minutes. Participation is voluntary.[1]

[1] "National Electronic Health Records Survey," Centers for Disease Control and Prevention (CDC), March 14, 2024. Available online. URL: www.cdc.gov/nchs/nehrs/index.html. Accessed September 24, 2024.

Section 7.4 | Mental Health Data and Research Methodologies in Childhood

THE IMPORTANCE OF CHILDREN'S MENTAL HEALTH

Mental health is an important part of children's overall health and well-being. It includes children's mental, emotional, and behavioral well-being and affects how they think, feel, and act. Additionally, mental health plays a role in how children handle stress, relate to others, and make healthy choices.

Mental disorders among children are characterized by serious changes in the way they typically learn, behave, or handle their emotions, leading to distress and difficulties in daily functioning. Among the more common mental disorders that can be diagnosed in childhood are attention-deficit/hyperactivity disorder (ADHD), anxiety, and behavior disorders.

ASSESSING MENTAL HEALTH IN CHILDREN

There are different ways to assess mental health and mental disorders in children. The Centers for Disease Control and Prevention (CDC) uses surveys, such as the National Survey of Children's Health, to describe the presence of positive indicators of children's mental health and to understand the number of children diagnosed with mental disorders and whether they received treatment. In these surveys, parents report on indicators of positive mental health for their child and any diagnoses their child has received from a health-care provider.

FACTS ABOUT MENTAL HEALTH IN U.S. CHILDREN

National data on positive mental health indicators that describe mental, emotional, and behavioral well-being for children are limited. Based on the available data:

- **Indicators of positive mental health are present in most children**. Parents reported in 2016–2019 that their child mostly or always showed:
  - affection (97.0%), resilience (87.9%), positivity (98.7%), and curiosity (93.9%) among children aged 3–5 years

- curiosity (93.0%), persistence (84.2%), and self-control (73.8%) among children aged 6–11 years
- curiosity (86.5%), persistence (84.7%), and self-control (79.8%) among children aged 12–17 years

FACTS ABOUT MENTAL DISORDERS IN U.S. CHILDREN

- **ADHD, anxiety problems, behavior problems, and depression are the most commonly diagnosed mental disorders in children.** Estimates for "ever having a diagnosis" among children aged 3–17 years from 2016 to 2019 are as follows:
  - ADHD: 9.8 percent (approximately 6.0 million)
  - anxiety: 9.4 percent (approximately 5.8 million)
  - behavior problems: 8.9 percent (approximately 5.5 million)
  - depression: 4.4 percent (approximately 2.7 million)
- **Some of these conditions commonly occur together.** For example, among children aged 3–17 years in 2016:
  - having another mental disorder was most common in children with depression: about three in four children with depression also had anxiety (73.8%), and almost one in two had behavior problems (47.2%)
  - among children with anxiety, more than one in three also had behavior problems (37.9%), and about one in three also had depression (32.3%)
  - for children with behavior problems, more than one in three also had anxiety (36.6%), and about one in five also had depression (20.3%)
- **Depression and anxiety have increased over time.**
  - The rates of "ever having been diagnosed with either anxiety or depression" among children aged 6–17 years increased from 5.4 percent in 2003 to 8 percent in 2007 and to 8.4 percent in 2011–2012.
  - The rates for "ever having been diagnosed with anxiety" increased from 5.5 percent in 2007 to 6.4 percent in 2011–2012.

- The rate for "ever having been diagnosed with depression" did not change significantly between 2007 (4.7%) and 2011–2012 (4.9%).
- **Among adolescents, depression, substance use, and suicide are significant concerns.** In 2018–2019, among adolescents aged 12–17 years reporting on the past year:
  - 5.1 percent had a major depressive episode
  - 36.7 percent had persistent feelings of sadness or hopelessness
  - 4.1 percent had a substance use disorder
  - 1.6 percent had an alcohol use disorder
  - 3.2 percent had an illicit drug use disorder
  - 18.8 percent seriously considered attempting suicide
  - 15.7 percent made a suicide plan
  - 8.9 percent attempted suicide
  - 2.5 percent made a suicide attempt requiring medical treatment
- **Treatment rates vary among different mental disorders.** Among children aged 3–17 years in 2016, treatment rates for mental health conditions were as follows:
  - Nearly 8 in 10 children (78.1%) with depression received treatment.
  - 6 in 10 children (59.3%) with anxiety received treatment.
  - More than 5 in 10 children (53.5%) with behavior disorders received treatment.
- **Mental, behavioral, and developmental disorders begin in early childhood.** One in six U.S. children aged 2–8 years (17.4%) had a diagnosed mental, behavioral, or developmental disorder.
- **The prevalence of mental disorders changes with age.**
  - Diagnoses of ADHD, anxiety, and depression become more common with increased age.
  - Behavior problems are more common among children aged 6–11 years than in younger or older children.
- **Many family, community, and health-care factors are related to children's mental health.**

  - Among children aged 2–8 years, boys were more likely than girls to have a mental, behavioral, or developmental disorder.
  - Among children living below 100 percent of the federal poverty level, more than one in five (22%) had a mental, behavioral, or developmental disorder.
  - Age and poverty level affected the likelihood of children receiving treatment for anxiety, depression, or behavior problems.
- **Adverse childhood events (ACEs) are associated with children's physical and mental health.** In 2016–2019, among children aged 6–17 years, the following trends were observed:
  - Children who experienced discrimination based on race or ethnicity had higher percentages of one or more physical health conditions (37.8% versus 27.1%) and one or more mental health conditions (28.9% versus 17.8%).
  - Racial/ethnic discrimination was almost seven times as common among children with three other adverse childhood experiences (ACEs) compared to those with no other ACEs.

RESEARCH ON CHILDREN'S MENTAL HEALTH IN THE COMMUNITY

The Project to Learn About Youth—Mental Health (PLAY—MH) analyzed information collected from four communities. The focus was on studying ADHD and other externalizing and internalizing disorders, as well as tic disorders in school-aged children. The purpose was to learn more about public health prevention and intervention strategies to support children's health and development.

Study questions included:

- What percentage of children in the community had one or more externalizing, internalizing, or tic disorders?
- How frequently did these disorders appear together?
- What types of treatment were children receiving in their communities?

RESEARCH ON PREVALENCE

Health-care providers, public health researchers, educators, and policymakers can obtain information about the prevalence of children's mental health disorders from various sources. Data sources, such as national surveys, community-based studies, and administrative claims data (such as health-care insurance claims), utilize different study methods and provide distinct types of information, each with its advantages and disadvantages:

- **National surveys have large sample sizes needed to create estimates at the national and state levels.** However, they generally rely on parents' reports of their child's diagnosis, meaning that health-care providers must provide accurate diagnoses and parents must accurately recall them.
- **Community-based studies allow children to observe their symptoms, allowing for the identification of children who may not have been diagnosed or who do not have the correct diagnosis.** However, these studies are typically conducted in small geographic areas, so findings may not be representative of other communities.
- **Administrative claims consist of extensive datasets containing diagnosis and treatment information directly from providers, which allows for tracking changes over time.** However, diagnoses or services that would not be reimbursed by specific health insurance may not be recorded in the data.

Using multiple data sources together provides more comprehensive information, enabling descriptions of:

- children with diagnosed conditions compared to children with the same symptoms but who are not diagnosed
- differences between populations with or without health insurance
- changes in estimates for mental health disorders over time

NATIONAL DATA ON CHILDREN'S MENTAL HEALTH

A comprehensive report from the Centers for Disease Control and Prevention (CDC), *Mental Health Surveillance Among Children—United States, 2013–2019*, described federal efforts to monitor mental disorders and presented estimates of the number of children with specific mental disorders, as well as positive indicators of mental health. The report was developed in collaboration with the Substance Abuse and Mental Health Services Administration (SAMHSA), the National Institute of Mental Health (NIMH), and the Health Resources and Services Administration (HRSA). It represents an update to the first-ever cross-agency children's mental health surveillance report in 2013.

The goal is to build on the strengths of federal agencies serving children with mental disorders to:

- develop better methods to document how many children have these disorders
- gain a better understanding of the consequences of mental disorders
- inform the needs for treatment and intervention strategies
- promote the mental health of children

This report is an important step toward recognizing the consequences of childhood mental disorders and developing a public health approach to address children's mental health.[1]

[1] "Data and Statistics on Children's Mental Health," Centers for Disease Control and Prevention (CDC), March 8, 2023. Available online. URL: www.cdc.gov/childrensmentalhealth/data.html. Accessed September 24, 2024.

Chapter 8 | Ethical and Cultural Considerations in Health Research

Chapter Contents

Section 8.1 | Ethical Standards for Informed Consent in Research

OVERVIEW OF INFORMED CONSENT REGULATIONS

The U.S. Department of Health and Human Services (HHS) regulations at 45 CFR Part 46 for the protection of human subjects in research require that an investigator obtain the legally effective informed consent of the subject or the subject's legally authorized representative, unless (1) the research is exempt under 45 CFR 46.101(b); (2) the institutional review board (IRB) finds and documents that informed consent can be waived (45 CFR 46.116(c) or (d)); or (3) the IRB finds and documents that the research meets the requirements of the HHS Secretarial waiver under 45 CFR 46.101(i) that permits a waiver of the general requirements for obtaining informed consent in a limited class of research in emergency settings. When informed consent is required, it must be sought prospectively and documented to the extent required under HHS regulations at 45 CFR 46.117.

ETHICAL FOUNDATIONS OF INFORMED CONSENT

The requirement to obtain the legally effective informed consent of individuals before involving them in research is one of the central protections provided under the HHS regulations at 45 CFR Part 46. This requirement is founded on the principle of respect for persons, one of the three ethical principles governing human subjects research described in the Belmont Report. The principle of respect for persons requires that individuals be treated as autonomous agents and that the rights and welfare of persons with diminished autonomy be appropriately protected. The Belmont Report states that an autonomous agent is "an individual capable of deliberation about personal goals and of acting under the direction of such deliberation." Respect for persons requires that prospective research subjects "be given the opportunity to choose what shall or shall not happen to them" and thus necessitates adequate standards for informed consent.

KEY FEATURES OF THE INFORMED CONSENT PROCESS

The informed consent process involves three key features:

1. disclosing to potential research subjects information needed to make an informed decision
2. facilitating the understanding of what has been disclosed
3. promoting the voluntariness of the decision about whether or not to participate in the research

Informed consent must be legally effective and prospectively obtained. HHS regulations at 45 CFR 46.116 and 45 CFR 46.117 describe the informed consent requirements.

THE ROLE OF INVESTIGATORS IN INFORMED CONSENT

The informed consent process is the critical communication link between the prospective human subject and an investigator, beginning with the initial approach of an investigator to the potential subject (e.g., through a flyer, brochure, or any advertisement regarding the research study) and continuing until the completion of the research study. For the purposes of the HHS regulations at 45 CFR Part 46, "investigators" are individuals who conduct human subjects research projects, including those directly involved in seeking the voluntary informed consent of potential subjects. Investigators can include physicians, scientists, nurses, administrative staff, teachers, and students, among others.

COMMUNICATION METHODS IN INFORMED CONSENT

The informed consent process should be an active process of sharing information between the investigator and the prospective subject. The exchange of information between the investigator and prospective subjects can occur via one or more of the following modes of communication, among others: face-to-face contact, mail, telephone, video, or fax. Prospective subjects should be provided with ample opportunity to ask questions and seek clarification from the investigator. The prospective subjects should be in a position to freely decide whether to initially enroll in the research or later withdraw or continue participating in the research. The informed consent process should ensure that all critical information about a study is completely disclosed and that prospective subjects or their legally authorized representatives adequately understand the research so that they can make informed choices.

DOCUMENTATION AND ONGOING CONSENT

The procedures used in seeking and obtaining informed consent should be designed to communicate with the subject population in terms that they can understand. Information about a research project must be presented in such a way that enables each person to voluntarily decide whether or not to participate as a research subject. Thus, the information must be conveyed in language understandable to those being asked to participate as subjects in the research (45 CFR 46.116).

For most research, informed consent is documented using a written document that provides key information regarding the research. The consent form is intended, in part, to provide information for the potential subject's current and future reference and to document the interaction between the subject and the investigator. However, even if a signed consent form is required, it alone does not constitute an adequate consent process. The informed consent process is an ongoing exchange of information between the investigator and the subject and could include, for example, the use of question-and-answer sessions, community meetings, and videotape presentations. In all circumstances, however, individuals should be provided with an opportunity to have their questions and concerns addressed on an individual basis.

REVISIONS AND IRB APPROVAL

The consent process and its documentation should be revised when deficiencies in its accuracy or completeness are noted, when new information about reasonably foreseeable risks and potential benefits becomes available, or when other additional information becomes known that will improve the consent process. Such revisions must be reviewed and approved by an IRB prior to the revised consent being utilized except when necessary to eliminate apparent immediate hazards to subjects (45 CFR 46.103(b)(4)).

LEGAL EFFECTIVENESS OF INFORMED CONSENT

Informed consent is legally effective if it is both obtained from the subject or the subject's legally authorized representative and documented in a manner consistent with the HHS protection of human subjects regulations and with applicable laws of the jurisdiction in which the research is conducted. In general terms, the regulations stipulate that an investigator should seek consent only under circumstances that provide the prospective subject or the legally authorized representative sufficient opportunity to consider whether to participate and that minimize the possibility of coercion or undue influence. The information provided should be in language that is understandable to the subject or the representative. No informed consent, whether oral or written, may include any exculpatory language.

It is important to note that the informed consent requirements in the regulations are not intended to preempt any applicable federal, state, or local laws that require additional information to be disclosed for consent to be legally effective (45 CFR 46.116(e)).

IRB WAIVERS OF INFORMED CONSENT

The HHS regulations allow the IRB to waive the requirement for obtaining informed consent or parental permission or to approve a consent procedure that leaves out or alters some or all of the elements of informed consent otherwise required under 45 CFR 46.116(a) and (b).

Waiving the requirement for obtaining informed consent or parental permission means that the IRB has determined that investigators need not obtain the subjects' informed consent to participate in research. For example, some research about natural behavior may require that subjects be unaware that the research is taking place. The IRB can only approve such research if it meets the criteria for a waiver of informed consent under HHS regulations and for approving research according to 45 CFR 46.111.

An IRB may approve research for which some or all of the elements of informed consent at 45 CFR 46.116(a) and (b) have been altered or for which some elements have been left out. For example, some research designs require that subjects be left unaware of the particular purpose of the research because the subjects' responses might be biased if they know in advance what the investigators are seeking. Such research designs do not preclude offering potential subjects some information about the research and giving them the opportunity to decide whether to participate. The IRB may approve such research in which investigators will leave out or alter elements of informed consent, so long as the research meets the criteria for approving research in 45 CFR 46.111 and the research meets the criteria specified in the HHS regulations for leaving out or altering those elements.[1]

Section 8.2 | **Cultural Competence in Health Services**

Nowhere are the divisions of race, ethnicity, and culture more sharply drawn than in the health of the people in the United States. Despite recent progress in overall national health, disparities continue in the incidence of illness and death among African Americans, Latino/Hispanic Americans, Native Americans, Asian Americans, Alaska Natives, and Pacific Islanders compared with the U.S. population as a whole.

Health and human service organizations are recognizing the need to enhance services for culturally and linguistically diverse populations. Providing culturally and linguistically appropriate health-care services requires an understanding of cultural competence.

WHAT IS CULTURAL COMPETENCE?

Cultural and linguistic competence is a set of congruent behaviors, attitudes, and policies that come together in a system, agency, or among professionals that enables effective work in cross-cultural situations. "Culture" refers to integrated patterns of human behavior that include the language, thoughts, communications, actions, customs, beliefs, values, and institutions of racial, ethnic, religious,

[1] "Informed Consent FAQs," U.S. Department of Health and Human Services (HHS), April 9, 2019. Available online. URL: www.hhs.gov/ohrp/regulations-and-policy/guidance/faq/informed-consent/index.html. Accessed September 25, 2024.

or social groups. "Competence" implies having the capacity to function effectively as an individual and an organization within the context of the cultural beliefs, behaviors, and needs presented by consumers and their communities.

Cultural competence requires that organizations:

- **Define values and principles.** Organizations must demonstrate behaviors, attitudes, policies, and structures that enable effective cross-cultural work.
- **Build capacity for diversity.** They should value diversity, conduct self-assessments, manage the dynamics of difference, acquire and institutionalize cultural knowledge, and adapt to the diversity and cultural contexts of the communities they serve.
- **Integrate these elements into policy.** Organizations should incorporate these components in all aspects of policymaking, administration, practice, and service delivery, systematically involving consumers, key stakeholders, and communities.

Cultural competence is a developmental process that evolves over an extended period. Both individuals and organizations are at various levels of awareness, knowledge, and skills along the cultural competence continuum.

Cultural competence is the integration and transformation of knowledge about individuals and groups of people into specific standards, policies, practices, and attitudes used in appropriate cultural settings to increase the quality of services and produce better outcomes.

PRINCIPLES OF CULTURAL COMPETENCE

- Define culture broadly.
- Value clients' cultural beliefs.
- Recognize complexity in language interpretation.
- Facilitate learning between providers and communities.
- Involve the community in defining and addressing service needs.
- Collaborate with other agencies.
- Professionalize staff hiring and training.
- Institutionalize cultural competence.

Improved quality of care is the outcome measure that indicates whether implementing training programs, policies, and culturally or linguistically appropriate standards makes a difference. A new trend in the literature suggests that using cultural competency in a focused or strategic way can be a helpful adjunct to the quality improvement process. For example, if a program wants to analyze patterns of broken appointments, it might examine variables such as age, gender, or race/ethnicity. If the analysis reveals that adolescents have the highest rate of broken appointments, the program can target specific strategies for this group. Does the clinic need to have weekend hours when teens can more easily slip away from home? Would providing free transportation or reminder calls from caseworkers help? Does the provider reflect a youth-sensitive approach to the clinic's client base?

CULTURAL COMPETENCE, AWARENESS, AND SENSITIVITY

Cultural competence emphasizes the idea of effectively operating in different cultural contexts and altering practices to reach different cultural groups. Cultural knowledge, sensitivity, and awareness do not include this concept. Although they imply an understanding of cultural similarities and differences, they do not include action or structural change.

CROSS-CULTURAL COMPETENCE IN HIV/AIDS CARE

The National Academy of Medicine report *Unequal Treatment: Confronting Racial and Ethnic Disparities in Health Care* states:

> *...racial and ethnic minorities tend to receive a lower quality of health care than nonminorities, even when access-related factors, such as patients' insurance status and income, are taken into account.*

These findings and others like them are not news to people concerned with the care of individuals living with human immunodeficiency virus (HIV) disease. Study after study has demonstrated unequal access to care and poorer health outcomes among certain segments of the HIV-positive population. For example, analysis of data from the HIV Cost and Services Utilization Study revealed that compared with nonminorities, women and African Americans with HIV disease who are receiving care are less likely to receive antiretroviral therapy, protease inhibitors, and prophylaxis for pneumocystis pneumonia. These disparities remained even after adjusting for gender, age, education, and insurance coverage. Follow-up in 1997 revealed improvements, but African Americans and Hispanics were still only about half as likely as whites to participate in HIV clinical trials or to receive experimental medicines. Other minorities were also less likely than whites to receive experimental treatment.

Disparities in access to quality care extend beyond race and gender to other segments of the population that are often marginalized. For example, HIV-infected injection drug users are less likely to receive antiretroviral therapy than non-drug users. It follows that disparities in access to quality HIV care are related to disparities in survival, which have been reflected in AIDS (acquired immunodeficiency syndrome) mortality data for some time.

Being competent in cross-cultural functioning means learning new patterns of behavior and effectively applying them in appropriate settings. For HIV/AIDS prevention and treatment to succeed, the special needs and life contexts of those who are marginalized because of race, ethnicity, socioeconomic status (SES), sexual orientation, age, or gender must be sensitively addressed. Cultural competence must be demonstrated not only by intervention programs and staff but also by surveillance staff, researchers (and their investigations), as well as by those delivering prevention services, care, and treatment programs to those who are HIV-infected.[1]

Section 8.3 | Enhancing Cultural Competence for Effective Health-Care Decisions

Providers striving to deliver high-quality care to all patients understand that cultural factors influence patients' health beliefs, behaviors,

---

[1] National Prevention Information Network (NPIN), "Cultural Competence in Health and Human Services," Centers for Disease Control and Prevention (CDC), June 24, 2024. Available online. URL: https://npin.cdc.gov/pages/cultural-competence-health-and-human-services. Accessed September 24, 2024.

and responses to medical issues. This information provides guidance for how to consider cultural differences as you build effective relationships with your patients during shared decision-making.

LEARN HOW TO INTERACT

- **Keep an open mind.** Remember that each patient has a unique set of beliefs and values, and they may not share yours.
- **Ask patients about their beliefs regarding their health condition.** For example, "What do you think caused the problem? What do you fear most about the sickness? Why do you think it started when it did?" This information will allow you to make the most of your interactions during shared decision-making. Recognize and understand that the meaning or value of health prevention, intervention, and treatment may vary greatly among cultures, specifically for behavioral health.
- **Attend cultural competence training at your organization or through a continuing education program.**
- **Be aware of your own culture and how that may affect how you communicate with your patients.**
- **Reach out to cultural brokers to help you learn more about the differences and similarities between cultures.** They can tell you how to better address the patients you serve regarding cultural appropriateness, beliefs about health, and barriers to communication. Cultural brokers might include health-care and social service workers and cultural group leaders. Ask them to suggest resources you can use to learn more about your patients' cultures.
- **Know what you do not know.** You will not be able to learn about every aspect of every patient's culture. Do not be afraid to let your patients know that you are unfamiliar with their culture. Invite them to explain what is important to them and how getting and staying well works in their community.

Keep in mind that culture is not homogenous. There is great diversity among individuals—even in the smallest cultural group.

Remember, culture changes over time, especially when one cultural group is exposed to and influenced by another culture.

PROVIDE CULTURALLY APPROPRIATE DECISION AIDS

- **Ask your patient about their learning preferences to help you present information better during shared decision-making.** Find out if your patient prefers for you to offer materials in print, video, or audio format. Ask your patient if they would like you to explain by talking, using a model, making a drawing, or demonstrating how to do something. You may find your patient wants you to present information in a variety of ways.
- **Use culturally relevant resources.** Ensure multimedia decision aids (videos, DVDs, CDs, audiotapes), other health resources for treatment, and other intervention materials reflect the cultures of the patients you serve.
- **Whenever possible, provide decision aids, treatment summaries, and educational materials that describe the risks and benefits of treatment options in a culturally relevant way.** The best decision aids meet cultural and health literacy or plain language standards.
- **Assess the quality of decision aids by using the International Patient Decision Aids Standards (IPDAS) Collaboration Criteria Checklist (http://ipdas.ohri.ca/index.html).**

PROVIDE QUALIFIED MEDICAL INTERPRETERS

- **Provide qualified medical interpreters for patients whose English proficiency is limited.** It is not advisable to use unqualified interpreters—such as a family member, friend, or unqualified staff member—and never to use a minor child to interpret. Using unqualified interpreters is more likely to result in misunderstandings and medical errors.
- **Expose cultural misunderstandings by asking patients to say in their own words what you have taught them.**

WORK TO BUILD TRUST

- **Show respect for your patients in culturally appropriate ways.** Make it clear that your role is to help them choose from among the options, not to make the decision for them.
- **Recognize that in many cultures, family members are deeply involved in health decisions.** Involve extended family members, when appropriate, in shared decision-making and when planning care.
- **Encourage patients to ask you questions.** Explain that asking questions is a good way to learn about health problems and treatment options. Say, "What questions do you have for me today?"
- **Choose signs, magazines, brochures, and other printed materials that reflect your patients' cultures.** This will help put them at ease.

Ensure comprehension by gently asking patients or family members to convey the information in their own words. Nodding and saying "yes" does not always mean comprehension has been achieved.[1]

Section 8.4 | Diversity and Inclusion in Clinical Trials

Our health is a combination of physical and mental well-being, which is affected by our behavior, biology, environment, societal policies, and, importantly, our lived experiences. The lived experiences of people in the United States vary based on their race and ethnicity, socioeconomic status (SES), geographic location, sexual orientation, gender identity, and other sociodemographic characteristics.

[1] Agency for Healthcare Research and Quality (AHRQ), "The SHARE Approach—Taking Steps toward Cultural Competence," U.S. Department of Health and Human Services (HHS), September 2020. Available online. URL: www.ahrq.gov/health-literacy/professional-training/shared-decision/tool/resource-7.html. Accessed September 25, 2024.

A clinical trial is a type of clinical research that evaluates the effects of intervention(s), including drugs, devices, surgeries, diets, behavioral approaches, and lifestyle interventions, on health-related biomedical or behavioral outcomes.

To account for the diverse lived experiences and exposures of various populations, clinical research should be appropriately inclusive of racial and ethnic minority groups, as well as other populations experiencing health disparities, including sexual and gender minority or socioeconomically disadvantaged populations.

WHY ARE CLINICAL TRIALS IMPORTANT?

Clinical trials can accomplish several objectives, including the following:

- determining if a new intervention is safe, works better, and/or has fewer side effects than an existing treatment or intervention
- examining ways to detect a disease early, when it is potentially more treatable, or ways to prevent a health problem altogether
- evaluating ways to improve the quality of life of people who have an illness or chronic medical condition
- testing behavioral, social, environmental, and structural interventions

Participating in clinical trials is voluntary. People volunteer to participate in clinical trials for a variety of reasons.

- One of the most common reasons is altruism—the opportunity to contribute to science and the common good and/or help those with similar health issues.
- People may volunteer when it allows them to receive an experimental intervention for a life-threatening or disabling disease where no standard treatments are available or have already been tried without success.
- New interventions (e.g., weight loss or tobacco cessation interventions) that have not yet been approved by the U.S. Food and Drug Administration (FDA) may be tested for common conditions to

understand if the intervention might help in situations where current treatments or interventions do not exist, do not work well, have unwanted side effects, or provide symptomatic relief but offer no cure.

THE IMPORTANCE OF DIVERSITY AND INCLUSION IN CLINICAL TRIALS

People may experience the same disease differently. It is essential that clinical trials include people with a variety of lived experiences and living conditions, as well as characteristics such as race and ethnicity, age, sex, and sexual orientation so that all communities can benefit from scientific advances.

Factors that can influence the risk and likelihood of developing a disease, experiencing a long-term health outcome, and responding to treatment include (but are not limited to):

- age
- biological sex
- pregnancy status
- life experiences (negatives, such as psychosocial stress and lack of basic resources, or positives, such as educational and employment opportunities)
- unhealthy behaviors (e.g., substance use, sedentary lifestyle, overeating, risky sexual activity)
- health-promoting behaviors (e.g., adequate sleep, obtaining recommended preventive services, physical activity, healthy eating)
- environmental conditions (e.g., pollution, access to health care or healthy foods, neighborhood segregation)
- genetic variation and geographic ancestry
- underlying medical problems or presence of comorbidities (i.e., additional diseases or conditions)

Historically, clinical trials did not always recruit participants who represented the people most affected by a particular disease, condition, or behavior. Often, these clinical trials relied almost exclusively on white male study participants. This shortcoming has created gaps in our understanding of diseases and conditions, preventive factors, and treatment effectiveness across populations. These gaps in knowledge can impede the quality of health-care decision-making, the ability to counsel people on ways to reduce their risk, optimal treatment responses, and even the development of more effective medications or interventions.

Clinicians and researchers should carefully consider the inclusion or exclusion criteria for their clinical trials. For example, a clinical trial excluding participants with high blood pressure or other comorbidities may end up excluding many people over 65 years old, who are more likely to have these conditions. The trial may then underrepresent certain groups in the study and make the results less applicable to groups that may benefit the most from the findings.

REAL-WORLD EXAMPLES OF THE NEED FOR INCLUSION IN CLINICAL TRIALS

COVID-19 Disparities

During the early stages of the pandemic, coronavirus 2019 (COVID-19) disproportionately affected racial and ethnic minority populations, including African-American, Hispanic/Latino, American Indian/Alaska Native, and Native Hawaiian and Pacific-Islander population groups, with increased cases, hospitalizations, and deaths.

It was critical that COVID-19 vaccine trials included sufficient representation across population groups to better understand vaccine effectiveness in populations who vary in environmental exposures and other lived experiences. By using inclusive recruitment practices in COVID-19 clinical trials, researchers have been able to show that vaccine safety and efficacy are similar across all racial and ethnic populations. Engaging diverse populations in planning and implementing such trials can also help increase public confidence that the vaccine is safe and effective.

Asthma Disparities

Asthma disparities are intricately linked with the environment. Living in a city may increase exposure to air pollution and the risk of developing asthma. Exposure to tobacco smoke, chronic social stress, or unhealthy diets may also influence asthma risk or severity. Thus, it is vital for clinicians and researchers to consider where patients live, what they eat, and how they feel—as well as characteristics such as race, ethnicity, socioeconomic status, and age—to get a more thorough understanding of their patients' experience with asthma symptoms and identify the best preventative strategies or treatment options.

INCLUSION OF SEXUAL AND GENDER MINORITY POPULATIONS

Until recently, health-care systems and epidemiological surveys often did not ask sexual orientation and gender identity questions to consider the inclusion of sexual and gender minority (SGM) individuals. This has made it difficult to know if people within SGM populations are represented in clinical research studies in significant numbers to make results representative for them. This lack of knowledge can influence patient-clinician communication and can result in fewer health screening or treatment opportunities.[1]

[1] "Diversity and Inclusion in Clinical Trials," National Institute on Minority Health and Health Disparities (NIMHD), January 12, 2024. Available online. URL: www.nimhd.nih.gov/resources/understanding-health-disparities/diversity-and-inclusion-in-clinical-trials.html. Accessed September 25, 2024.

Part 2 | Social Determinants of Health across Demographic Groups

Chapter 9 | The Role of Social Determinants in Public Health

Social determinants of health (SDOH) are the nonmedical factors that influence health outcomes. They are the conditions in which people are born, grow, work, live, and age. These forces and systems include a wide set of factors that shape daily life, such as:

- economic policies and systems
- development agendas
- social norms
- social policies
- political systems

The Centers for Disease Control and Prevention (CDC) has adopted this definition from the World Health Organization (WHO).

WHY ARE SOCIAL DETERMINANTS OF HEALTH IMPORTANT TO THE CDC?

Social determinants of health are one of three priority areas for Healthy People 2030, along with health equity and health literacy.

Healthy People 2030 sets data-driven national objectives in five key areas of SDOH:

- health-care access and quality
- education access and quality
- social and community context

- economic stability
- neighborhood and built environment

Some examples of SDOH included in Healthy People 2030 are safe housing, transportation, and neighborhoods; polluted air and water; and access to nutritious foods and physical health opportunities.

As the federal government's leading public health agency, the CDC has a unique role in contributing to work on SDOH.

WHY IS ADDRESSING SOCIAL DETERMINANTS OF HEALTH IMPORTANT FOR THE CDC AND PUBLIC HEALTH?

Addressing differences in SDOH accelerates progress toward health equity, a state in which every person has the opportunity to attain their highest level of health. SDOH have been shown to have a greater influence on health than either genetic factors or access to health-care services. For example, poverty is highly correlated with poorer health outcomes and a higher risk of premature death. SDOH, including the effects of centuries of racism, are key drivers of health inequities within communities of color. The effect is pervasive and deeply embedded in our society, creating inequities in access to a range of social and economic benefits—such as housing, education, wealth, and employment. These inequities put people at higher risk of poor health.

The CDC is coordinating efforts to focus its resources on the areas where federal public health investments can make the most difference. For example, the CDC's Racial and Ethnic Approaches to Community Health (REACH; www.cdc.gov/reach/php/about) focuses on reducing high rates of chronic diseases for specific racial and ethnic groups in urban, rural, and tribal communities. Since 1999, the program has worked across sectors in racial and ethnic minority communities to reduce tobacco use, improve access to healthy foods, change the built environment to promote physical activity, and connect people to clinical care.

PUBLIC HEALTH ACTIONS THAT AFFECT SOCIAL DETERMINANTS OF HEALTH

Public health organizations can take several actions to promote health and well-being, including the following:

Convene

Bring together community members and organizations to identify local concerns. The CDC has a long history of convening partners through national conferences, webinars, collaborative publications, and guideline development. The CDC also encourages other public health organizations to act as conveners by requiring coalition-building or community engagement activities in some funded projects.

Integrate

Collect and use multiple sources of data, including public health data, to help develop strategies for setting direction. For example, public health departments can provide GIS maps of community needs and assets based on CDC PLACES data (www.cdc.gov/places/index.html) and environmental justice data (www.cdc.gov/environmental-health-tracking/php/data-research/environmental-justice.html).

Influence

Lead approaches to develop policies and solutions or leverage funding through various mechanisms to implement and expand priority actions. For example, when CDC Director Rochelle Walensky announced that racism is a public health threat in 2021, it reinforced actions that communities were already taking and supported many others as they took subsequent actions.

Contribute to Big Changes

Collaborate with others to find innovative solutions and implement them. For example, an LA County public health initiative resulted in a ban on menthol cigarettes.

CDC'S SOCIAL DETERMINANTS OF HEALTH FRAMEWORK

In fall 2021, CDC leadership started an agencywide process to build and expand cross-cutting efforts to address SDOH. This effort was led by the National Center for Chronic Disease Prevention and Health Promotion (NCCDPHP) and resulted in a framework of six pillars:

1. **Data and surveillance**. Embed a consistent SDOH approach to standardization, collection, analysis, and dissemination of data across the agency.
2. **Evaluation and evidence building**. Advance evaluation and build evidence for strategies that address SDOH to reduce disparities and promote health equity.
3. **Partnerships and collaboration**. Establish criteria, actionable steps, and strategies for partnerships, collaborations, and relationships that result in improved health outcomes over the long term.
4. **Community engagement**. Foster meaningful, sustained community engagement across all phases of CDC intervention planning and implementation.
5. **Infrastructure and capacity**. Strengthen and sustain infrastructure such as workforce, training, and access to financial resources required to address SDOH and reduce health disparities.
6. **Policy and law**. Identify evidence, tools, and resources to enhance communication with policymakers and other stakeholders about policies that affect SDOH.

The CDC is using this framework to help agency leadership make decisions about where to invest SDOH resources.[1]

---

[1] "Social Determinants of Health (SDOH)," Centers for Disease Control and Prevention (CDC), January 17, 2024. Available online. URL: www.cdc.gov/about/priorities/why-is-addressing-sdoh-important.html. Accessed September 25, 2024.

Chapter 10 | Socioeconomic Status and Health

Chapter Contents

Section 10.1 | The Effect of Socioeconomic Status on Health Outcomes

HOW SOCIOECONOMIC STATUS INFLUENCES HEALTH

"Socioeconomic status" refers to the absolute or relative levels of economic resources, power, and prestige closely associated with the wealth of an individual, community, or country. It is a multidimensional construct comprising multiple factors, such as income, education, employment status, and others.

Low socioeconomic status is associated with a higher risk of developing and dying from cardiovascular disease (CVD). Specifically, the American Heart Association notes that income level, educational attainment, and employment status at the individual and neighborhood levels are consistently associated with CVD in high-income countries. Socioeconomic factors can affect health status directly at the individual level and can also influence broader household, neighborhood, or community-level characteristics, which can then affect health.

Socioeconomic factors affect one's ability to engage in health activities, afford medical care and housing, and manage stress. For example, employment provides income, which enables access to housing, education, childcare, food, medical care, and other needs. At the community level, lower-income neighborhoods are less likely to have access to high-quality health care.

Socioeconomic factors can also interact with or confound relationships between other variables and health. For example, the combined effects of socioeconomic status and race/ethnicity or sex can influence health differently across different groups.

EDUCATION

Education is strongly associated with life expectancy and morbidity. Research has shown that by the age of 25, a college graduate is expected to live a decade longer than a high school dropout. Many studies, including a meta-analysis of hypertension research, have observed that lower levels of education are associated with a greater risk of CVD than higher levels of education.

Education plays an important role in health through its influence on multiple socioeconomic factors, such as employment, income, and other economic opportunities. Individuals with lower levels of educational attainment are more likely to lack sociopolitical power and economic resources, leading to adverse occupational, residential, and recreational conditions associated with negative health consequences. These adverse conditions lead to differential exposures to stressors (such as unemployment, crime, and violence) and fewer resources (such as recreation and physical activities) to cope with the accumulation of stressors that contribute to a greater risk of hypertension.

EMPLOYMENT STATUS

Employment status (whether an individual is working to earn wages) is consistently identified as an indicator of socioeconomic status strongly associated with health outcomes. Employment status affects health through both physical and psychosocial pathways. Employees may be exposed to hazardous physical, chemical, or biological agents from the occupational setting. Unstable employment can lead to loss of compensation and employee benefits (such as health insurance), creating psychosocial stress. In the United States, health care is accessed predominantly through employer-sponsored health insurance plans. Loss of employment results in loss of health-care insurance coverage. The short-term unemployed tend to experience the greatest barriers to health-care access, as they may not be able to take advantage of public benefits. Even in cases where individuals may qualify for public insurance assistance through the Consolidated Omnibus Budget Reconciliation Act (COBRA) or other public programs, the copayments and deductibles are often too costly for those with reduced or no steady income. The long-term unemployed and those unable to work may be eligible for Medicaid. Those who are self-employed also experience barriers to health care, as individual insurance plans are often not as comprehensive as employer-sponsored plans. Barriers to health-care access due to loss of employer-sponsored health coverage are associated with reduced health-care utilization and unfavorable health outcomes.

INCOME

The relationship between income and health is well established. Households with incomes below the federal poverty level (annual income thresholds set by the federal government to determine financial eligibility criteria) have high levels of illness and premature mortality. Individuals with lower incomes lack economic resources, resulting in social disadvantage, poor education, poor working conditions, housing insecurity, and residence in unsafe neighborhoods. These negative environmental and psychosocial factors affect behavioral and physiological pathways that have proximal effects on health, including increased morbidity and mortality. The United States has experienced a rise in income inequality, with widening racial gaps in wealth. For every dollar of wealth that white households have, Asian, Hispanic/Latino, and Black/African-American households have 83, 7, and 6 cents, respectively. It is estimated that in the United States, the gap in life expectancy between the top 1 percent of wage earners and the bottom 1 percent is 14.6 years for men and 10.1 years for women. Moreover, over the past few decades, life expectancy has increased among the wealthiest 20 percent, while the remaining 80 percent have not experienced any gains in life expectancy.

One study found that the richest 20 percent of study participants had healthier levels of biomarkers for cardiovascular disease, including body mass index (BMI), systolic blood pressure, and high-density lipoproteins, relative to the poorest 80 percent of participants. Individuals with lower incomes are more likely to experience adverse psychosocial factors that can induce a physiological stress response, resulting in higher circulating levels of catecholamines, cortisol, and blood pressure.

FOOD INSECURITY

"Food insecurity," defined as the disruption of food intake or eating patterns due to insufficient financial resources and other resources, is closely related to income and unemployment and is widely recognized as a risk factor for chronic diseases, such as hypertension, coronary heart disease (CHD), hepatitis, stroke, cancer, asthma, diabetes, arthritis, chronic obstructive pulmonary disease (COPD), and kidney disease. In 2020, it was estimated that 10.5 percent of U.S. households experienced food insecurity, and the prevalence of food insecurity was notably higher for single-parent households and Black/African-American and Hispanic/Latino households.

Food insecurity negatively affects health through three pathways: unhealthy nutrition; monetary trade-offs; and psychological distress. First, food insecurity is associated with poorer diet quality, which may lead to metabolic dysregulation, fat accumulation, or insulin resistance. Second, relieving and mitigating food insecurity often involves monetary trade-offs between purchasing food or medication that may severely limit people's ability to manage chronic conditions properly. Third, food insecurity is strongly associated with psychological distress, lower self-efficacy, and depressive symptoms, triggering physiological stress responses (such as elevated cortisol levels) and unhealthy coping behaviors (such as excessive drinking, smoking, and drug use).

HOUSING INSECURITY

"Housing insecurity" is commonly defined as high housing costs relative to income, but it has also been used as an umbrella term to describe multiple housing issues, such as poor housing quality, unstable occupancy, overcrowding, and unsafe neighborhoods. Housing-insecure adults are more likely to delay medical care and utilize emergency care, have poorer health-care access, experience adverse mental health outcomes, and have a higher prevalence of substance use than individuals with stable housing.

Eviction and foreclosure are associated with exposure to violence, depression, anxiety, increased alcohol use, psychological distress, and suicide.

Homeownership offers stable housing and is a protective factor for mental health. Homeowners report higher self-esteem and happiness than renters and people experiencing housing insecurity, results that could reduce stress. Homeownership is also associated with better psychosocial health, such as a reduced burden of depression.[1]

---

[1] "Socioeconomic Factors," Centers for Disease Control and Prevention (CDC), September 1, 2023. Available online. URL: www.cdc.gov/dhdsp/health_equity/socioeconomic.htm. Accessed September 25, 2024.

Section 10.2 | Economic Burden of Health Disparities in the United States

Research shows that the economic burden of health disparities in the United States remains unacceptably high. The study, funded by the National Institute on Minority Health and Health Disparities (NIMHD), part of the National Institutes of Health (NIH), revealed that in 2018, racial and ethnic health disparities cost the U.S. economy $451 billion, a 41 percent increase from the previous estimate of $320 billion in 2014. The study also finds that the total burden of education-related health disparities for individuals with less than a college degree in 2018 reached $978 billion, about two times greater than the annual growth rate of the U.S. economy in 2018.

This study is the first to estimate the total economic burden of health disparities for five racial and ethnic minority groups nationally and for all 50 states and the District of Columbia using a health equity approach. The health equity approach sets aspirational health goals that all populations can strive for, derived from the Healthy People 2030 goals. It establishes a single standard that can be applied to the nation and each state, and for all racial, ethnic, and education groups. It is also the first study to estimate the economic burden of health disparities by educational levels as a marker of socioeconomic status.

ECONOMIC BURDEN BY RACIAL AND ETHNIC MINORITY GROUPS

National Estimates

- Most of the economic burden for racial and ethnic disparities was borne by the Black/African-American population (69%) due to the level of premature mortality.
- Native Hawaiian/Pacific-Islander ($23,225) and American Indian/Alaska Native ($12,351) populations had the highest economic burden per person.
- Most of the economic burden was attributed to premature deaths for Native Hawaiian/Pacific-Islander (NHPI; 90%), Black/African-American (77%), and American Indian/

Alaska Native (AI/AN; 74%) populations. For Asian (55%) and Hispanic/Latino (43%) populations, most of the burden was from excess medical care costs and lost labor market productivity, respectively.

State Estimates

- The five states with the highest burden of racial and ethnic health inequities were among the most populous and diverse: Texas ($41 billion), California ($40 billion), Illinois ($29 billion), Florida ($27 billion), and Georgia ($21 billion).
- Black/African-American people had the highest economic burden of racial and ethnic health inequities in most states (33 states), followed by Hispanic/Latino (9 states), American Indian/Alaska Native (8 states), and Native Hawaiian/Pacific-Islander (1 state) individuals.
- The burden of racial and ethnic health disparities relative to each state's GDP varied from 0.14 percent (Vermont) to 8.89 percent (Mississippi). In 2018, 17 states had a burden higher than the annual growth rate of the U.S. economy.

ECONOMIC BURDEN BY EDUCATIONAL LEVELS

National Estimates

- Per person, adults with a high school diploma had the highest burden ($9,982), followed closely by adults with less than a high school diploma ($9,467) and then adults with some college ($2,028).
- Although most of the burden of education-related health inequities was borne by adults with a high school diploma or GED (61%), a disproportionate share was borne by adults with less than a high school diploma or GED—they were only 9 percent of the population but bore 26 percent of the burden.
- Across all educational levels, most of the burden was attributable to premature deaths (66%), followed by lost labor market productivity (18%) and excess medical care costs (16%).

State Estimates

- Per person, the economic burden of health disparities varied substantially across states by educational levels. For adults with less than a high school diploma, the burden ranged from $3,152 (California) to $21,372 (Kentucky). For adults with a high school diploma, it ranged from $6,201 (West Virginia) to $25,555 (South Carolina), and for adults with some college, it ranged from $1,072 (Illinois) to $8,374 (South Carolina).
- In 31 states, adults with less than a high school diploma/ GED had the highest economic burden of education-related health inequities. In 20 states, the burden was greatest among adults with a high school diploma/ GED. Adults with some college had the lowest burden of education-related health inequities in all 50 states and the District of Columbia.
- The burden of education-related health inequities relative to each state's GDP varied from 1.90 percent (District of Columbia) to 18.29 percent (South Carolina). In 2018, 46 states had a burden higher than the annual growth rate of the U.S. economy.

While the economic burden of racial and ethnic and education-related health disparities is significant, the researchers noted that the burden could be reduced if investments are made to address structural contributors to known inequities, including racism and socioeconomic inequalities. They also recommended that federal and state health policymakers and offices of minority health could use these estimates to inform areas where policies and programs are most needed to address health inequities.[1]

[1] News and Events, "NIH-Funded Study Highlights the Financial Toll of Health Disparities in the United States," National Institutes of Health (NIH), May 16, 2023. Available online. URL: www.nih.gov/news-events/news-releases/nih-funded-study-highlights-financial-toll-health-disparities-united-states. Accessed September 25, 2024.

Section 10.3 | **Employment Status and Health-Care Access**

A study from the National Institute for Occupational Safety and Health (NIOSH) found that health-care access and other health-related needs in the United States differ by employment status. Researchers evaluated these needs among people who were employed for wages, self-employed, short-term unemployed (less than a year), long-term unemployed (a year or more), or unable to work. Health-care access was most problematic among the short-term unemployed. The prevalence of adverse health outcomes increased with the length of unemployment status and was highest among respondents unable to work. The study was published online November 8, 2021, in the *American Journal of Industrial Medicine*.

"In the U.S. healthcare system, healthcare access is closely linked to work, with the majority of working-age adults having employer-sponsored insurance," said Sharon Silver, epidemiologist and lead author of the study. "While people with very low incomes and a subset of those unable to work are eligible for public benefits, the short-term unemployed may have difficulty accessing both employer-sponsored and public benefits."

NIOSH researchers used the 2018–2019 Behavioral Risk Factor Surveillance System data, which includes self-reported information on a variety of topics, including employment and health, from 278,424 respondents aged 25–54 in the United States who met the study definition. Researchers assessed health-care access and use, health-related behaviors, and health outcomes by employment status.

Short-term unemployed respondents were most likely to face challenges accessing health care. Researchers found this group was least likely to have health insurance or a personal health-care provider. Nearly one in three short-term unemployed respondents reported needing to see a doctor in the past year but were unable to due to costs. Self-employed individuals had gaps in health-care use and were least likely to have had a routine checkup within the last year.

Respondents who were unemployed were more likely to report adverse health outcomes than those employed or self-employed. The prevalence of fair or poor self-rated health, poor physical and mental health, obesity, and 10 chronic health conditions increased from the short-term unemployed to the long-term unemployed and was highest among those unable to work. More than half of the respondents who were unable to work reported having fair or poor general health, poor physical health, or diagnosed depression. Additionally, almost half of those unable to work had obesity, and more than 40 percent reported poor mental health, hypertension, and high cholesterol.

"Employment is a social determinant of health and a health equity issue, particularly given the link between employment and healthcare access. Our research shows that unemployed individuals and those unable to work face increased challenges when it comes to healthcare access and health outcomes," said Silver. "Addressing access to affordable healthcare and other resources is key to preventing health declines that may hinder re-employment, particularly among the short-term unemployed."[1]

Section 10.4 | **Understanding Employment Discrimination and Your Rights**

The U.S. Equal Employment Opportunity Commission (EEOC) enforces federal laws that protect you from discrimination in employment. If you believe you have been discriminated against at work or in applying for a job, the EEOC may be able to help.

WHO IS PROTECTED?

- employees (current and former), including managers and temporary employees
- job applicants
- union members and applicants for membership in a union

[1] National Institute for Occupational Safety and Health (NIOSH), "NIOSH Study Examines Relationship between Employment Status, Healthcare Access, and Health Outcomes," Centers for Disease Control and Prevention (CDC), November 18, 2021. Available online. URL: www.cdc.gov/niosh/updates/upd-11-18-21.html. Accessed September 25, 2024.

WHAT ORGANIZATIONS ARE COVERED?

- most private employers
- state and local governments (as employers)
- educational institutions (as employers)
- unions
- staffing agencies

WHAT TYPES OF EMPLOYMENT DISCRIMINATION ARE ILLEGAL?

Under the EEOC's laws, an employer may not discriminate against you, regardless of your immigration status, on the bases of:

- race
- color
- religion
- national origin
- sex (including pregnancy, childbirth, and related medical conditions, sexual orientation, or gender identity)
- age (40 and older)
- disability
- genetic information (including employer requests for, or purchase, use, or disclosure of genetic tests, genetic services, or family medical history)
- retaliation for filing a charge, reasonably opposing discrimination, or participating in a discrimination lawsuit, investigation, or proceeding
- interference, coercion, or threats related to exercising rights regarding disability discrimination or pregnancy accommodation

WHAT EMPLOYMENT PRACTICES CAN BE CHALLENGED AS DISCRIMINATORY?

All aspects of employment, including:

- discharge, firing, or layoff
- harassment (including unwelcome verbal or physical conduct)

- hiring or promotion
- assignment
- pay (unequal wages or compensation)
- failure to provide reasonable accommodation for a disability, pregnancy, childbirth, or related medical condition, or a sincerely held religious belief, observance, or practice
- benefits
- job training
- classification
- referral
- obtaining or disclosing genetic information of employees
- requesting or disclosing medical information of employees
- conduct that might reasonably discourage someone from opposing discrimination, filing a charge, or participating in an investigation or proceeding
- conduct that coerces, intimidates, threatens, or interferes with someone exercising their rights or someone assisting or encouraging someone else to exercise rights regarding disability discrimination (including accommodation) or pregnancy accommodation

WHAT CAN YOU DO IF YOU BELIEVE DISCRIMINATION HAS OCCURRED?

Contact the EEOC promptly if you suspect discrimination. Do not delay, because there are strict time limits for filing a charge of discrimination (180 or 300 days, depending on where you live/work). You can reach the EEOC in any of the following ways:

- Submit an inquiry through the EEOC's Public Portal: https://publicportal.eeoc.gov/Portal/Login.aspx.
- Call:
  - Toll-free: 800-669-4000.
  - Teletypewriter (TTY): 800-669-6820.
  - American Sign Language (ASL) video phone: 844-234-5122.

- Visit an EEOC Field Office (information at www.eeoc.gov/field-office).
- Email: info@eeoc.gov.

Additional information about the EEOC, including details about filing a charge of discrimination, is available at www.eeoc.gov.[1]

Section 10.5 | Managing Occupational Hazards and Health Risks

A systematic approach to hazard identification and control is essential for promoting workplace safety and health. Engaging workers and implementing effective controls can significantly reduce the risk of injuries and create a safer working environment.

HAZARD IDENTIFICATION AND ASSESSMENT

One of the "root causes" of workplace injuries, illnesses, and incidents is the failure to identify or recognize hazards that are present or that could have been anticipated. A critical element of any effective safety and health program is a proactive, ongoing process to identify and assess such hazards.

To identify and assess hazards, employers and workers should take the following steps:

- Collect and review information about the hazards present or likely to be present in the workplace.
- Conduct initial and periodic workplace inspections to identify new or recurring hazards.
- Investigate injuries, illnesses, incidents, and close calls/near misses determining the underlying hazards, their causes, and safety and health program shortcomings.

[1] "Know Your Rights: Workplace Discrimination Is Illegal," U.S. Equal Employment Opportunity Commission (EEOC), June 27, 2023. Available online. URL: www.eeoc.gov/know-your-rights-workplace-discrimination-illegal. Accessed September 25, 2024.

- Group similar incidents and identify trends in injuries, illnesses, and reported hazards.
- Consider hazards associated with emergency or nonroutine situations.
- Determine the severity and likelihood of incidents that could result from each hazard identified and use this information to prioritize corrective actions.

Some hazards, such as housekeeping and tripping hazards, can and should be fixed as they are found. Fixing hazards on the spot emphasizes the importance of safety and health and takes advantage of a safety leadership opportunity.

HAZARD PREVENTION AND CONTROL

Effective controls protect workers from workplace hazards, help avoid injuries, illnesses, and incidents, minimize or eliminate safety and health risks, and help employers provide workers with safe and healthful working conditions.

To effectively control and prevent hazards, employers should take the following actions:

- Involve workers, who often have the best understanding of the conditions that create hazards and insights into how they can be controlled.
- Identify and evaluate options for controlling hazards using a "hierarchy of controls."
- Use a hazard control plan to guide the selection and implementation of controls, and implement controls according to the plan.
- Develop plans with measures to protect workers during emergencies and nonroutine activities.
- Evaluate the effectiveness of existing controls to determine whether they continue to provide protection or whether different controls may be more effective. Review new technologies for their potential to be more protective, more reliable, or less costly.[1]

---

[1] "Recommended Practices for Safety and Health Programs," Occupational Safety and Health Administration (OSHA), October 18, 2016. Available online. URL: www.osha.gov/safety-management. Accessed September 25, 2024.

Chapter 11 | Strategies for Advancing Educational Equity

The U.S. Department of Education (ED) has included the following five strategies in its 2023 Equity Action Plan Update to help achieve educational equity and excellence:

STRATEGY 1:
Improve College Access, Affordability, and Degree Completion for Underserved Students to Increase Economic Mobility

The ED aims to address barriers to college access, affordability, and completion by supporting colleges to enroll more students from underserved groups, including students of color, students from low-income backgrounds, students who are English learners, and others. This strategy seeks to raise graduation rates and close graduation rate gaps for these student populations and offer affordable credentials of value that lead to careers offering economic mobility.

STRATEGY 2:
Implement Maintenance of Equity Requirements to Ensure Historically Underserved Students Have Equitable Resources for Learning Recovery

The ED aims to ensure that school districts serving historically underserved student groups, including students of color, students from low-income backgrounds, students who are English learners, students experiencing homelessness, and others, have the resources they need to support learning recovery. This includes the allocation of $122 billion in American Rescue Plan (ARP) funds for Title I schools and the ARP's Maintenance of Equity requirements to protect high-poverty schools from reductions in state and local education funding. More specifically, the Maintenance of Equity provision safeguards high-poverty school districts and schools from disproportionate reductions in per-pupil state and local education aid.

STRATEGY 3:
Address Inequities Faced by Justice-Impacted Individuals by Expanding Access to Postsecondary Learning Opportunities That Improve Outcomes for Communities and Reduce Recidivism Rates

The ED aims to ensure that our society is more just and equitable by supporting better opportunities for education during periods of incarceration and post-release. Current initiatives are set to improve the well-being of incarcerated individuals and increase successful reentry outcomes, smoothing pathways to further education, increasing workforce readiness and engagement, and reducing recidivism and preventing crime. This includes partnerships between institutions of higher education, correctional agencies, accrediting agencies, and community-based organizations.

STRATEGY 4:
Advance Equity in and through Career and Technical Education

The ED aims to invest in career and technical education to create new and inclusive pathways to well-paying jobs and upward mobility. This includes leveraging data to promote strategies that reduce segregation by gender, race, and ethnicity in high school Career and Technical Education (CTE) programs.

STRATEGY 5:
Increase Mental Health Resources with an Emphasis on Underserved Communities, from the Historic Legislation and Funding Provided by the Bipartisan Safer Communities Act

The ED aims to address the youth mental health crisis by working with states to support local educational agencies (LEAs) with high rates of poverty through three top priorities:

1. Increasing the skills and knowledge of existing school personnel to support the mental health needs of students.
2. Increasing the supply of mental health professionals who can work with students.
3. Increasing funding through the Medicaid program to support school health services, including mental health services.[1]

[1] "Equity Action Plan Update," U.S. Department of Education (ED), 2023. Available online. URL: www2.ed.gov/documents/equity/2023-equity-plan.pdf. Accessed September 27, 2024.

Chapter 12 | **Childhood and Early Development**

Chapter Contents

HEALTHY EATING IN CHILDHOOD AND ADOLESCENCE

Healthy eating in childhood and adolescence is important for proper growth and development and to prevent various health conditions. The *Dietary Guidelines for Americans, 2020–2025* recommends that people aged two years or older follow a healthy eating pattern that includes:

- a variety of fruits and vegetables
- whole grains
- fat-free and low-fat dairy products
- a variety of protein foods
- oils

These guidelines also recommend that individuals limit calories from solid fats (major sources of saturated and *trans* fatty acids) and added sugars and reduce sodium (salt) intake. Unfortunately, most children and adolescents do not follow the recommendations in the *Dietary Guidelines for Americans.*

BENEFITS OF HEALTHY EATING

Healthy eating can help individuals achieve and maintain a healthy body weight, consume important nutrients, and reduce the risk of developing health conditions such as:

- high blood pressure (HBP)
- heart disease
- type 2 diabetes
- cancer
- osteoporosis
- iron deficiency
- dental caries (cavities)

DIET AND ACADEMIC PERFORMANCE

- Schools are in a unique position to provide students with opportunities to learn about and practice healthy eating behaviors.

- Eating a healthy breakfast is associated with improved cognitive function (especially memory), reduced absenteeism, and improved mood.
- Adequate hydration may also improve cognitive function in children and adolescents, which is important for learning.

EATING BEHAVIORS OF YOUNG PEOPLE

- Between 2001 and 2010, consumption of sugar-sweetened beverages among children and adolescents decreased, but these beverages still account for 10 percent of total caloric intake.
- Between 2003 and 2010, total fruit intake and whole fruit intake among children and adolescents increased. However, most youth still do not meet fruit and vegetable recommendations.
- Empty calories from added sugars and solid fats contribute to 40 percent of daily calories for children and adolescents aged 2–18 years, affecting the overall quality of their diets. Approximately half of these empty calories come from six sources: soda, fruit drinks, dairy desserts, grain desserts, pizza, and whole milk. Most youth do not consume the recommended amount of total water.[1]

Section 12.2 | **Reducing Health Disparities in Early Childhood Development**

THE IMPORTANCE OF EARLY CHILDHOOD DEVELOPMENT

Research suggests that many disparities in overall health and well-being are rooted in early childhood. Stressors in early childhood can disrupt neurologic, metabolic, and immunologic systems, leading to

[1] "Childhood Nutrition Facts," Centers for Disease Control and Prevention (CDC), August 5, 2022. Available online. URL: www.cdc.gov/healthyschools/nutrition/facts.htm. Accessed September 25, 2024.

poorer developmental outcomes. However, consistent, responsive caregiving relationships and supportive community and health-care environments promote an optimal trajectory. The first eight years of a child's life build a foundation for future health and life success. Thus, the cumulative and lifelong effect of early experiences, both positive and negative, on a child's development can be profound.

Although the health, social service, and education systems that serve young children and their families provide opportunities to support responsive relationships and environments, efforts by these systems are often fragmented due to restrictions that limit the age groups they can serve and the types of services they can provide. Integrating relationship-based prevention and intervention services for children early in life, when the brain is developing most rapidly, can optimize developmental trajectories. By promoting collaboration and data-driven intervention activities, public health can play a critical role in both the identification of at-risk children and the integration of systems that support healthy development. These efforts can address disparities by reducing barriers that might prevent children from reaching their full potential.

DEVELOPMENTAL TRAJECTORIES

Healthy child development includes not only physical developmental domains but also emotional, behavioral, cognitive, language, and general learning competencies. The human brain undergoes rapid growth during childhood, driven in part by a child's acquisition and integration of skills across many developmental domains. Development in all domains is finely integrated across neural circuitry, allowing for more complex learning and tasks over time. Skill acquisition depends on children being ready to learn and can be envisioned as a developmental trajectory.

Exposure to adversity and stressors such as poverty, lack of safety and stability in the home environment, and lack of access to quality early education can negatively affect a child's development. These exposures can lead to an "at-risk or vulnerable" trajectory and, in severe cases, a "delayed or disordered" trajectory. Conversely, protective factors provided in a child's home or community environment, such as consistent and responsive caregiving relationships and coordinated health care and other services, can reduce and even ameliorate the effect of adverse circumstances, allowing children to reach or return to a healthy trajectory.

Chronic stressors in early childhood, such as poverty, can have cumulative lifetime effects on learning, earnings, and health. Language differences associated with socioeconomic status have been documented as early as age 18 months. Vocabulary skills by age 3 years predict third-grade reading, which in turn predicts high school graduation rates. High school graduates achieve increased earning potential and are less likely to have chronic diseases, such as diabetes, chronic pain, and symptoms of mental disorders than non-graduates. High school graduates are also more likely to report good health and visit a health professional, important markers of positive health outcomes.

IDENTIFYING VULNERABLE CHILDREN AND INFORMING ACTION

Screening, early identification, and linkage to services can prevent vulnerable children (i.e., children at risk for or with a developmental delay) from progressing to levels of higher risk. For disadvantaged groups, early intervention can yield the greatest social and economic returns. For example, an economic analysis of two similar early childhood interventions for socioeconomically disadvantaged children, the Carolina Abecedarian Project and the Carolina Approach to Responsive Education, identified a 7.3 benefit/cost ratio and a 13.7 percent rate of return per annum when examining the long-term health, crime reduction, educational, and employment benefits of program participation.

Public health surveillance data characterize population-level effects and can be used to inform public health action. For example, recent analyses identified treatment patterns for young children with attention-deficit/hyperactivity disorder (ADHD) that were not aligned with the American Academy of Pediatrics' (AAP) recommendations. These data have led to collaborations to:

- increase awareness of recommendations for behavior therapy before medication for preschool children
- increase available behavioral therapy options for providers and families

- inform state and local decision-makers about best practices. Surveillance data continue to inform and monitor the effect of these collaborations and other early childhood initiatives

Screening measures inclusive of social determinants of health provide opportunities for strengthening protective factors through family, community, and health-care connections. Public health activities to improve early detection and referral to treatment include the Early Hearing Detection and Intervention programs to identify hearing loss in infants; online tools developed by CDC and AAP for identifying motor delays; and Learn the Signs. Act Early for children with or at risk for developmental disabilities. These tools leverage state, provider, and family-level actions to reduce the time to diagnosis and initiation of services.

INTEGRATING SUPPORT SERVICES FOR VULNERABLE CHILDREN AND THEIR FAMILIES

Many service agencies work to support optimal child development, but many have specific age requirements (e.g., early intervention, preschool, or school age) or provide specific types of services (e.g., developmental, health, social welfare, or educational). Too often, vulnerable children are identified but do not meet strict criteria for services of the agencies contacted, leaving them without needed services. An example of a program that has reduced service gaps by integrating available services for children is Help Me Grow. Help Me Grow serves as a centralized point of entry for both state- and community-based services where families of vulnerable children are matched to service agencies that offer the support they need. Through a single information line, vulnerable children who are likely to meet eligibility criteria are linked to publicly funded early intervention services, preschool special education services, and interventions for children with special health-care needs. Vulnerable children at risk due to environmental or biological factors but who do not meet eligibility requirements for the described services are linked to other community-based programs and services through Help

Me Grow. In 2015 alone, Help Me Grow served 42,511 children and their families. Promising evaluation results have led some states to embed the Help Me Grow model within various federal initiatives, including the Health Resources and Services Administration's Maternal, Infant, and Early Childhood Home Visiting and Early Childhood Comprehensive Systems, and the Substance Abuse and Mental Health Services Administration's (SAMHSA) Project LAUNCH (Linking Actions for Unmet Needs in Children's Health) program.

INTEGRATING BEHAVIORAL AND PHYSICAL HEALTH

Behavioral health services can promote the health and development of children when high-quality services can be Accessed by the children who need them. Nationally representative data from 2011 to 2012 suggest that 15 percent of U.S. children aged two to eight years have a parent-reported mental, behavioral, or developmental disorder, and children living in small rural areas have a higher prevalence (19%) than children living in urban areas (15%). In 2012, nearly $14 billion in medical expenditures for mental disorders among children were spent across all payment types (private insurance, public insurance, out-of-pocket, and other); these costs were higher than those for any other health condition (e.g., chronic obstructive pulmonary disease (COPD) and asthma, trauma-related conditions, and acute respiratory infections). However, only an estimated 20 percent of children and youth with behavioral problems receive mental health services. In particular, children in rural communities often have less access to early childhood interventions and behavioral health care services, highlighting the need for behavioral health care in alternative settings and coordinated care solutions.

Mental, behavioral, and developmental disorders in young children have been associated with potentially modifiable family, community, and health-care factors. Two-generation approaches that support the health, educational achievement, economic self-sufficiency, and well-being of both children and their caregivers have indicated some beneficial effects on early childhood literacy and language development. Within primary care, screening and referral to appropriate services for maternal depression can support the parent-child relationship and enhance both child and maternal health. For children facing circumstances that put them at risk, such as poverty, enhancing these maternal-child protective factors might be particularly important for reducing the negative effects of stressors on long-term child health. Furthermore, pediatric primary care can expand beyond anticipatory guidance by promoting protective factors and resiliency through evidence-based interventions that address parental self-care, positive parenting strategies, and parent-child relationship building. By coordinating and integrating care across medical systems and community providers, the prevention- and patient-focused medical home (family-centered coordinated primary care) model promotes both behavioral and physical health.

PROMOTING SUPPORTIVE RELATIONSHIPS ACROSS MULTIPLE CONTEXTS

Early childhood objectives outlined in Healthy People 2020 highlight the need to support parents and caregivers, create supportive communities, increase access to high-quality health care, and increase the proportion of children ready for school in all domains of healthy development. Programs that create connections across early learning and home environments by supporting family engagement in learning have demonstrated positive effects on young children's academic success and development. However, gaps exist in access to high-quality early care and education, training, and evidence-based resources to support family engagement partnerships. A 2016 AAP policy statement aimed at ameliorating the health and developmental effects of poverty describes the importance of effective interventions and strategies focused on economic aid, access to comprehensive care coordination, early care and education, early identification of children and families in need of services, and promotion of protective factors through family support programs. The common thread for these approaches is the focus on both risk factors and protective factors for the entire family across multiple systems, not simply on the child with an identified condition in a single context.

IMPORTANCE OF INTEGRATION AND COLLABORATION

Early childhood represents a period of growth that lays the foundation for successful learning, development, and health; disparities emerge early and widen over time. Intervening in early childhood can prevent the development of diseases and disorders among at-risk and vulnerable children but will require collaboration. Strategies that foster consistent and responsive caregiving relationships and supportive environments can improve outcomes for both parent and child. Parents and early care providers can work together to provide responsive interactions and consistent environments that nurture the development of young children. Practitioners can screen and identify children early, promote family strengths, and refer to services before risks progress. States and communities can use surveillance data to drive action around early childhood investments. Partners within public health can use data-informed approaches to prevent health disparities by facilitating service linkages across health, social, and educational systems. Timely referral and better-integrated services might help children at low or moderate risk reach their full potential by returning to healthy developmental trajectories.[1]

[1] "CDC Grand Rounds: Addressing Health Disparities in Early Childhood," Centers for Disease Control and Prevention (CDC), July 25, 2017. Available online. URL: www.cdc.gov/mmwr/volumes/66/wr/mm6629a1.htm. Accessed September 25, 2024.

Chapter 13 | **Integrating Services for Children and Families**

Chapter Contents

Section 13.1 | Linking Medicaid and Child Welfare Data to Improve Services and Outcomes

HEALTH NEEDS AND MEDICAID SERVICES FOR FAMILIES INVOLVED IN CHILD WELFARE SYSTEMS

Very little is known about the health needs of, and services used by, families involved in child welfare systems, particularly those services funded by Medicaid. Many families involved in child welfare throughout the process—including those whose only contact includes a child welfare referral—have low incomes and are eligible for Medicaid. Additionally, all children in foster care are eligible for Medicaid. The lack of research on this topic is, in large part, due to the limited availability of large-scale datasets on Medicaid use by families involved with child welfare systems. As child welfare programs focus more on preventing family removals, there is a need to coordinate information and operations across child welfare and Medicaid programs. Linking data among children and their caregivers who are served by both systems allows agencies, researchers, and other interested groups to identify opportunities to improve service provision and care coordination and potentially improve child and family outcomes. The U.S. Department of Health and Human Services's (HHS) Office of the Assistant Secretary for Planning and Evaluation (ASPE) has several efforts underway to support states in developing linked data to improve services to children and their families and provide policy-relevant research insights.

CCOULD PROJECT

The Child and Caregiver Outcomes Using Linked Data (CCOULD) project—funded by the Patient-Centered Outcomes Research Trust Fund—partnered with Florida and Kentucky to create a linked dataset of Medicaid and child welfare system data to facilitate research on the relationships between:

- child and caregiver Medicaid coverage and services
- child welfare services, health-care outcomes, and child welfare outcomes

CCOULD provided technical assistance to states in linking Medicaid administrative claims of children and their caregivers with case-level data from the child welfare system. It combined state-specific data into a deidentified dataset for secondary data analysis. The linked dataset contains information from both child welfare and Medicaid information systems on case demographics, medical diagnoses, services, outcomes, and other relevant information. These data can be obtained from the National Data Archive on Child Abuse and Neglect (www.ndacan.acf.hhs.gov/datasets/pdfs_user_guides/dataset272codebook.pdf).

Linked data on services from child welfare and Medicaid can be used to understand the effectiveness of interventions and improve coordination to address critical challenges faced by families at risk of child welfare system involvement.

CHILD WELFARE AND MEDICAID DATA LINKING LESSONS

This project identified lessons for federal and state agencies interested in similar linking projects. Key lessons learned include the following:

- States can benefit from support in navigating data governance.
    - Internal data-sharing initiatives within state agencies are subject to many legal, procedural, and regulatory requirements, which can slow down intra-agency data sharing.
    - Real and perceived regulatory and privacy concerns are equally important to address.
- Recruiting states for linked data efforts requires time and resources, engagement of multiple stakeholders, and adaptation to changing circumstances.
    - Honoraria or site payments may not fully offset the participation burden.
    - Memoranda of Understanding (MOUs) and Data Use Agreements (DUAs) must be site-specific, and negotiations can be time-consuming.

- Data-linking projects need to identify and plan for issues and gaps in data quality and documentation.
  - Documentation of state child welfare system variables could be more robust.
  - The lack of a family identifier in Medicaid claims and encounters data makes the identification of caregivers challenging.
  - Probabilistic matching can be more beneficial than deterministic matching to obtain as much linked data as possible.
- States need support in strengthening and harmonizing data infrastructure on child welfare services.

USING THE CCOULD DATASET FOR RESEARCH

The ASPE is taking steps to facilitate researchers' use of the CCOULD data and has identified key research topics to be addressed using the CCOULD dataset:

- Understanding the use of Medicaid services for behavioral health services, in particular substance use disorder (SUD) treatment.
- Learning how SUD services relate to services provided by child welfare systems.
- Gaining an understanding of how they relate to parent and child health and stability outcomes.
- Allowing testing of the effectiveness of new interventions to provide treatment and recovery services.

Additionally, ASPE has partnered with the Institute for Research on Poverty at the University of Wisconsin–Madison to establish a Research Consortium on Child Welfare Outcomes and Medicaid Utilization. The consortium will host regular meetings of invited researchers using the CCOULD dataset to align research studies, share lessons about working with the data, improve technical documentation, increase exposure to the utility of the dataset, and generate findings to support patient-centered outcomes research.

CHILDREN INITIATIVE

The Child Welfare and Health Infrastructure for Linking and Data Analysis of Resources, Effectiveness, and Needs (CHILDREN) Initiative, in partnership with Mathematica, builds on the lessons of CCOULD to link child welfare and Medicaid data, and also supports states in developing analytics to advance key policy priorities. CHILDREN's objectives include:

- Conduct feasibility studies to determine states' or municipalities' readiness and infrastructure to develop data systems with linked records from Medicaid and public child welfare agencies.
- Develop publicly available datasets and data systems with linked records from Medicaid and public child welfare agencies for children and parents or caregivers involved in both systems.
- Use linked records to (a) increase analytic opportunities to help better understand and improve child welfare operations, services, outcomes, and health services delivered to children and parents in the child welfare system; and (b) develop, pilot, and implement models to support oversight of prevention and congregate care services.
- Document lessons learned on linking data across the agencies.

Initial data linking work is expected to be complete by the end of 2025, with additional analytic tasks finishing in 2027.[1]

[1] Office of the Assistant Secretary for Planning and Evaluation (ASPE), "Improving Services for Children and Families through Linked Child Welfare and Medicaid Data," U.S. Department of Health and Human Services (HHS), July 2024. Available online. URL: https://aspe.hhs.gov/sites/default/files/documents/2b365e17ca982c2646074c184af1fae3/improving-services-children-families-data.pdf. Accessed September 26, 2024.

Section 13.2 | **Strategies for Successful Human Services Integration in Child Welfare**

The Office of the Assistant Secretary for Planning and Evaluation (ASPE) in the U.S. Department of Health and Human Services (HHS) has been working with researchers, human services agency leaders, and people with lived experience to visualize, describe, and document models of primary prevention within human services, including the prevention of child maltreatment.

To support this goal, ASPE contracted with Mathematica and the Center for the Study of Social Policy (CSSP) to conduct case studies of innovative prevention approaches that integrate human services. The brief highlights initiatives from this *Case Studies in Supporting Prevention Through Program Integration* project that used service integration and agency collaboration to achieve the following goals:

1. Increase protective factors.
2. Prevent child maltreatment and reduce substantiated reports.
3. Prevent homelessness among youth aging out of foster care.

Although these initiatives were geographically diverse and provided a range of services for the populations they served, their collective experiences pointed to four key themes for successful human services integration to prevent child welfare system involvement.

THEME 1:
Involve Community Members and Organizations in Planning, Designing, and Implementing an Integrated Services Approach

Involving residents, community leaders, and community-based organizations in developing and implementing their approaches helped sites build buy-in for services and ensured that the supports met community needs and reflected community and cultural values. Four sites had formal processes for community engagement.

- Families First DC (FFDC) used community members' feedback to develop a culturally resonant ongoing survey for family assessments. Each FFDC Family Success Center had a Community Advisory Council that met every month to assess emergent community needs and brainstorm services to meet them.

THEME 2:
Focus on Establishing Trust and Relationships with Families They Serve to Repair Harm

Sites emphasized the importance of developing relationships and promoting trust and safety for families. Staff from four sites noted that some families had a deep mistrust of services or programs associated with child welfare agencies due to a legacy of deficit-based service delivery and family separation. To remedy this mistrust, states (1) partnered with community-based organizations (CBOs) that community members trusted, (2) kept support services as distinct and stand-alone from child welfare as possible, and (3) oriented services around strengthening families and building on their assets and resources.

- In the Maine Foster Youth to Independence (FYI) initiative, the local housing authority was supposed to receive referrals of youth exiting foster care from the state child welfare agency. However, many youth did not want to continue contact or communication with the child welfare agency. FYI partnered with a trusted youth homeless shelter to identify youth eligible for the program.

THEME 3:
Use a Person-Centered Approach to Implement Services

A person-centered approach focuses on meeting families where they are to address their expressed needs and goals and prevent them from falling into crises or deeper involvement in the child welfare system. Four sites employed service navigators or case managers who worked individually with participants to assess their interests and goals and connect them with partners who could help them achieve those goals.

- Boulder County IMPACT Partnership used a care coordination team to help families receive appropriate support, such as Medicaid, and access the right systems based on their needs.

Five sites also provided concrete support to address families' individual urgent needs, prevent crises, and enable them to work on their goals. These supports included vouchers and gift cards to pay for rent and utilities, diapers and baby formula, groceries and cleaning supplies, and personal hygiene products, as needed by particular families.

- The Ohio Children's Trust Fund provided a $500 gift card to families participating in an evidence-based home visiting program.

THEME 4:
Braid Flexible Funding Sources to Respond to Communities' Varied Needs

The study sites were creative in braiding federal, state, and local funds to offer a holistic set of services to participants. For state-led initiatives, braiding happened at the state level, enabling community-based staff to focus on families' and individuals' needs, rather than tracking allowable services.

Georgia State of Hope used Community-Based Child Abuse Prevention (CBCAP) and Promoting Safe and Stable Families (PSSF) funds to make small grants—typically under $50,000—to local organizations. To braid the funding sources at the state level, staff in the Georgia Division of Child and Family Services matched the services that State of Hope grantees provided with eligible services that CBCAP and PSSF fund.[1]

---

[1] Office of the Assistant Secretary for Planning and Evaluation (ASPE), "Integrating Services to Strengthen Children, Youth, and Families and Prevent Involvement in the Child Welfare System," U.S. Department of Health and Human Services (HHS), July 2024. Available online. URL: https://aspe.hhs.gov/sites/default/files/documents/974d57d73a04f3d0ebf4bde2436efd1a/Prevention-Child-Welfare-Brief.pdf. Accessed September 25, 2024.

Section 13.3 | Strategic Framework for Addressing Youth Mental Health Disparities

The National Institute of Mental Health (NIMH) initiated the Strategic Framework for Addressing Youth Mental Health Disparities with the overarching goal of advancing scientific knowledge that can inform policies and practices to reduce mental health disparities in youth by 2031.

THE STRATEGIC FRAMEWORK COMPONENTS

The NIMH seeks to achieve progress in these components by supporting workforce development and research and through outreach and collaboration with various stakeholders. Under each component, examples of potential actions toward progress and metrics to assess progress are presented. These examples are not exhaustive and will be updated and refined as progress is made.

Component 1: Addressing Knowledge Gaps and Expanding Research Opportunities

The NIMH will encourage a full and diverse range of research—including basic science, translational science, and services and implementation research—focused on youth mental health disparities through the development of new initiatives and the publication of new funding opportunities. These efforts will promote mental health equity by supporting research on ways to decrease risk, increase resilience and protective factors, improve access to and utilization of quality care, and improve outcomes of treatment and services among populations negatively affected by mental health disparities.

The NIMH can take various actions to address knowledge gaps and expand research opportunities, including the following efforts:

- Support research to elucidate the mechanisms of action of social determinants of mental health, how they can be modified, and how they drive risk of, resilience to, and protection from the development of mental illnesses.

- Support research to identify and understand contextualizing factors, including environmental and historical factors, their influence on biology, emotion, cognition, and behavior, and how they mediate mental health disparities.
- Support research on how local, state, and federal policies, laws, and regulations affect social determinants of mental health, mental health service delivery, and outcomes among youth from populations affected by mental health disparities.
- Support research on variation in biological and genomic processes within and among diverse populations and settings historically underrepresented in genetics research.
- Support research, including longitudinal studies, to understand and measure how childhood experiences confer resilience to or risk for mental illnesses and suicidal thoughts and behaviors in youth from populations affected by mental health disparities.
- Support research to improve the specificity of biomarkers and the accuracy of culturally appropriate diagnostic assessments (including risk calculators) for youth from populations affected by mental health disparities.
- Support the development and validation of culturally appropriate preventive interventions, including systems-level approaches (e.g., in classrooms, schools, communities), for youth and parents from populations affected by mental health disparities.
- Support the optimization of existing evidence-based approaches to minimize bias in diagnosis and treatment, and to improve continuity of care and mental health outcomes for youth from populations affected by mental health disparities.
- Support research to address co-occurring mental illnesses in youth with intellectual and developmental disabilities, including youth intersecting with other high-risk groups.

- Support research to improve implementation and availability of mental health prevention and treatment interventions and services, as well as programs to support youth and family functioning within youth-serving institutions (e.g., educational settings, community-based after-school programs, faith-based programs, child welfare programs, and juvenile justice settings).
- Support research that uses innovative assessment and analytic methods to examine subpopulations and low base-rate behaviors and to address complex, multimodal datasets.
- Support translational research on developing, testing, and implementing prevention and treatment interventions relevant to communities affected by health disparities across a range of ages (e.g., infancy through young adulthood).
- Support research from collaborative teams that include community partners to ensure the outcomes and interpretation of the research reflect the priorities of the population participating in the research.
- Support research to develop targeted interventions by examining risk and resilience within populations affected by youth mental health disparities.

To estimate progress in addressing knowledge gaps and expanding research opportunities, the NIMH could examine:

- notices of special interest (NOSIs) focused on youth mental health disparities
- funding opportunity announcements (FOAs) to address youth mental health disparities
- grants funded on interventions targeting youth mental health disparities
- bibliometrics of NIMH-supported publications (e.g., relative citation ratios)
- advances related to improving suicide risk prevention and detection among youth from populations affected by mental health disparities

- advances related to improving access, engagement, and effectiveness of evidence-based mental health treatment and services for youth from populations affected by mental health disparities
- advances related to the effect of laws, policies, and structural determinants of health on youth from populations affected by mental health disparities

Component 2: Extending and Supporting Stakeholder Engagement

The NIMH will engage in outreach, collaboration, and dissemination efforts with youth with mental illnesses and their families, those with interest in or affected by youth mental health disparities, and those with research expertise. Stakeholders include, but are not limited to: patients, families, people with lived experience, mental health researchers and trainees, other scientists, a range of federal agencies within and outside the Department of Health and Human Services (HHS), policymakers, non-governmental organizations, educational organizations such as colleges and universities, health-care service administrators and payors, clinical care providers, and members of the public. Stakeholder engagement plays an important role in inspiring innovations in science, ensuring the public health relevance of research, encouraging the uptake of evidence-based practices and interventions, decreasing stigma and stereotyping, promoting responsible interpretation and communication of research findings, and increasing overall acceptability of mental health treatments and services, along with public awareness—thus strengthening the public health effect of research.

While the NIMH maintains longstanding relationships with numerous stakeholders, additional efforts to include a diversity of perspectives in mental health research will enhance relationships with researchers and populations affected by health disparities and increase the effect of NIH-supported scientific discoveries. Engagement helps to avoid "othering" and reinforcing stereotypes about youth and families affected by racial and ethnic health disparities.

Examples of NIMH actions to extend and support stakeholder engagement may include the following efforts:

- Seek sustained engagement with stakeholders to inform the NIMH's strategies for supporting research that addresses youth mental health disparities.
- Disseminate information about NIMH-supported advances in research on reducing youth mental health disparities.
- Facilitate outreach through professional society and advocacy group meetings to build networking opportunities, connect scientists and community members, and exchange information about the needs of individuals and communities, obstacles to research, and emerging research opportunities related to youth mental health disparities.
- Publish via the NIMH website and social media channels educational materials tailored for families and youth from groups with mental health disparities.
- Encourage NIMH-supported researchers to partner with communities in the development of their research projects, including but not limited to community-based participatory research.
- Promote collaborations across NIH Institutes, Centers, and Offices (ICOs; e.g., NICHD, NIMHD, the Office of Behavioral and Social Sciences Research (OBSSR)) and with other HHS agencies (e.g., Centers for Medicare & Medicaid Services (CMS), Substance Abuse and Mental Health Services Administration (SAMHSA), Indian Health Service (IHS)) to understand where the gaps in knowledge exist and how to widely implement evidence-based practices.

To estimate progress in stakeholder engagement, the NIMH could examine:

- NIMH-initiated public meetings and outreach activities about strategies for reducing youth mental health disparities

- NIMH staff attendance at scientific meetings that cover topics related to youth mental health disparities
- NIMH data reports related to youth mental health disparities in response to requests from public policymakers
- stakeholder engagement with public-facing NIMH messages and educational resources related to youth mental health disparities
- investigator-initiated applications incorporating community engagement
- collaborations addressing youth mental health disparities across NIH ICOs (e.g., NICHD, NIMHD, OBSSR) and with other HHS agencies (e.g., CMS, SAMHSA, IHS)

Component 3: Growing the Youth Mental Health Disparities Research Workforce

The NIMH will promote and support the growth and retention of a diverse research workforce, including those well-trained in youth mental health disparities research. To achieve this, the NIMH will support a range of research training and career development programs and funding opportunities to build, enhance, and sustain pathways to independent research careers for youth mental health disparities researchers.

Examples of NIMH actions to grow the youth mental health disparities research workforce may include the following efforts:

- Promote the training, retention, mentoring, and career transition of investigators in the youth mental health disparities research workforce.
- Participate in cross-NIH programs that promote diversity and inclusivity of the workforce in biomedical research.
- Raise awareness among early-career investigators about the variety of positions that may be involved in youth mental health disparities research.
- Support training for investigators on minimizing bias and other research equity issues.

- Enhance technical assistance, outreach, and capacity-building support for Historically Black Colleges and Universities and other Minority Serving Institutions in applying for research funding, including, but not limited to, research focused on youth mental health disparities.
- Support the inclusion of diverse perspectives on peer review panels to better appreciate youth mental health disparities research topics.
- Support mechanisms that encourage institutions to diversify their student and faculty populations to enhance the participation and inclusion of individuals from groups affected by mental health disparities.

To estimate progress in growing the youth mental health disparities research workforce, the NIMH could examine:

- grants from early-stage investigators (ESIs) on topics related to youth mental health disparities
- individuals supported by NIMH research training and career development mechanisms studying topics related to youth mental health disparities
- NIMH-supported trainees and ESIs studying topics related to youth mental health disparities who successfully complete the career stage being supported (e.g., completion of pre- or post-doctoral training; transition from "K" award to independent research project grant)
- NIMH-supported trainees and ESIs studying topics related to youth mental health disparities who are successfully retained in the youth mental health disparities research workforce 5–10 years after initial NIMH support
- dissemination/reach of NIMH-supported technical assistance and research equity training resources to the youth mental health disparities research workforce[1]

[1] "NIMH Strategic Framework for Addressing Youth Mental Health Disparities," National Institute of Mental Health (NIMH), February 1, 2023. Available online. URL: www.nimh.nih.gov/health/publications/nimh-strategic-framework-for-addressing-youth-mental-health. Accessed September 25, 2024.

Chapter 14 | **Cultural Humility and Community Engagement in Global Public Health**

EMBRACING CULTURAL HUMILITY AND COMMUNITY ENGAGEMENT

Everyone who works cross-culturally and cross-linguistically will make mistakes. In a world with diverse cultures and languages, it is crucial to be flexible and take responsibility for mistakes. It is also important to learn and adapt as cultures and languages evolve. Doing so helps build trust and relationships that are key to effective global public health efforts.

Global public health professionals, programs, and related communications belong to evidence-based public health and scientific agencies. Professionals in science-based agencies should demonstrate humility by learning from mistakes and adapting their approaches. Rigorous evaluation and community feedback often lead to better outcomes.

CULTURAL HUMILITY

Cultural humility is active engagement in an ongoing process of self-reflection that informs a deeper understanding and respect for cultural differences. Increased cultural humility can lead to more culturally appropriate behaviors, programs, policies, practices, and services.

Increasing Cultural Humility

- **Examine your personal history, background, and social position.** Evaluate how the following factors affect your interpersonal relationships:
  - gender
  - ethnicity
  - socioeconomic status
  - profession
  - education
  - assumptions, values, beliefs, and biases
  - culture
- **Reflect on how your professional organization affects interactions and relationships with community members.** A health professional's affiliation with an organization can positively or negatively affect interactions and relationships. The organization's reputation, history, norms, and perceived power can influence how people perceive health professionals who represent that organization.
- **Understand and respect cultural differences.** To gain a deeper understanding and respect for cultural differences, practice:
  - active inquiry and reflection
  - openness to power-balanced relationships
  - appreciation of another person's or community's lived experience and social and cultural expertise
- **Recognize when you are not the expert.** Everyone has gaps in their experience and expertise. Be willing to learn from local people and communities about their experiences and practices. Avoid judgment as much as possible.

Implementing Cultural Humility

- **Emphasize mutually beneficial partnerships.** Global public health professionals should emphasize collaborative, mutually beneficial, and peer-to-peer approaches for solving shared challenges together.

Avoid the posture, framing, and language of hierarchy, patriarchy, supremacy, and saviorism.

- **Make findings and products accessible**. Make findings and final products accessible to the communities and collaborators involved in the research, programs, or initiatives. Offer communication products in local languages and beyond written text, such as verbal presentations, group meetings, individual discussions, and infographics.
- **Avoid perpetuating harmful hierarchies and supremacies**. Actively identify and avoid markers of hierarchy and supremacy that are often seen in the global public health sector. The markers noted below can occur across different forms of hierarchy and supremacy rooted in nationality and ethnicity, gender, income, education, ability, age, and sexual orientation.

COMMUNITY ENGAGEMENT

Global public health professionals should prioritize community engagement. Doing so builds foundational trust and relationships and strengthens collaboration. This helps ensure everyone involved has an equal opportunity to share their voices, opinions, or ideas for public health research, projects, and communications that affect their lives and livelihoods.

Community engagement leads to more effective, sustainable, locally appropriate, and community-owned communication, programs, partnerships, and research.

Leverage Existing Relationships

Leverage existing relationships with local partners and community members to proactively identify, listen to, and incorporate a range of people. This broader range of people will bring additional perspectives, experiences, and knowledge. Additional insights can benefit projects and programs throughout the planning, development, implementation, and evaluation phases.

If a relationship with the community does not yet exist, work with and follow the lead of trusted intermediaries who do have existing relationships.

Availability and Accessibility

Ensure platforms and safe spaces are available and accessible for people from all involved parties to raise their voices throughout the project. Ideally, each involved party should have equal speaking time during discussions. At each stage of the project, note who is or is not speaking and who was included or excluded.

- **Using the local language fosters inclusive engagement.** Global public health professionals who are not familiar with the local language should work closely with partners or translators who are fluent.
- **Identify if social or cultural norms prevent participation.** Identify whether any social or security constraints exist that could hinder community members' participation. If constraints exist, identify how engagement, planning, and implementation can be adapted. For example, some women might have limited mobility, farmers may be busy during the day, or seasonal workers may be unavailable at certain times of the year.
- **Ensure everyone can get the information that is shared.** Assess the appropriateness of descriptive video, closed captioning, teletypewriter (TTY), and other accommodations for individuals with disabilities. When these options are not available, consider recording or transcribing meetings and allowing members extra time to review materials. Translate materials if language barriers exist.

ACTIVE COMMUNITY PARTICIPATION

Ensure that communities are encouraged and have the opportunity to actively participate throughout the project. Community members should be actively engaged in designing, implementing, leading, evaluating, and improving the public health research, projects, and communications that affect them. Identify potential gaps in participation and implement the most inclusive processes possible before moving to the next stage. Ideally, community members should determine priorities and lead subsequent actions and initiatives.

If some participants are present during a discussion but are not active participants, consider whether any power dynamics affect their willingness to speak. For example, people perceived to be of a lower social caste may be unwilling, hesitant, or barred from speaking in front of those perceived to be of a higher social caste.

In some cases, it might be necessary to convene participants in separate groups. For example, a women's group and a men's group, or an adult group and an adolescent group, might need to meet separately.

Support People in Sharing Their Own Story

Especially for communication activities that involve storytelling, engage all parties to tell their own stories. Ensure that the overall narrative is from the community, not merely about the community.

The person with lived experience is the expert on their own story. Ideally, the power to write or dictate the story should rest with the person or community with lived experience. In such an arrangement, a professional communicator should be in a support role, offering input and advice as appropriate.

When a professional communicator is developing the story, use quotes and expand on the surrounding context. Focus the narrative and action on the person or community's own ideas about what is needed for them to live healthy and secure lives.

When storytelling across languages, ensure that translation is high quality so that key nuances are not lost. Ensure that stories incorporate a range of experiences to represent the diversity of the population.

Invite and Include Community Members in Research and Publications

Encourage and invite local partners to contribute as authors of research publications. Any authors from local institutions who contribute and meet authorship criteria must be included as authors in the final published version.

While abiding by institutional and journal authorship criteria, engage in open discussion to clarify contributions, negotiate authorship, and publish with an accurate and adequate order of authorship.

Encourage and promote local authors as first and senior authors. Local authors are often underrepresented in key authorship positions in literature about their own countries.[1]

[1] "Embracing Cultural Humility and Community Engagement," Centers for Disease Control and Prevention (CDC), May 15, 2024. Available online. URL: www.cdc.gov/global-health-equity/php/publications/cultural-humility.html. Accessed September 25, 2024.

Chapter 15 | **Social Cohesion and Community Engagement**

Chapter Contents

Section 15.1 | The Influence of Social Cohesion on Health Outcomes

Relationships are important for physical health and psychosocial well-being. Relationships are conceptualized through terms such as social cohesion, social capital, social networks, and social support. "Social cohesion" refers to the strength of relationships and the sense of solidarity among members of a community. One indicator of social cohesion is the amount of social capital a community has. Social capital deals with shared group resources, such as a friend-of-a-friend's knowledge of a job opening. Individuals have access to social capital through their social networks, which are webs of social relationships. Social networks are sources of multiple forms of social support, such as emotional support (e.g., encouragement after a setback) and instrumental support (e.g., a ride to a doctor's appointment). This summary will review the positive and negative health effects social cohesion has on a person's life.

SOCIAL CAPITAL AND HEALTH

Social capital is an important marker of social cohesion, and it has significant ramifications for health. For example, one study examined the link between four measures of social capital ("perceived fairness," "perceived helpfulness," "group membership," and "trust"), income inequality, and mortality. All four measures of social capital were found to be associated with mortality. They also found that the relationship between income inequality and mortality may be partially explained by reductions in social capital as income inequality increases.

COLLECTIVE EFFICACY

"Collective efficacy," an aspect of social capital and social cohesion, is grounded on mutual trust and describes a community's ability to create change and exercise informal social control (i.e., influence behavior through social norms). Collective efficacy is associated with better self-rated health, lower rates of neighborhood violence, and better access to health-enhancing resources such as medical care, healthy food options, and places to exercise. Social institutions such as religion and the family are common sources of social capital and social control, as well as social networks and social support.

SOCIAL NETWORKS AND HEALTH BEHAVIORS

Social networks spread social capital, but they can also spread health behaviors and outcomes, a phenomenon known as "social contagion." For example, if a person's friend, sibling, or spouse is obese, the person's likelihood of also becoming obese increases. Similar patterns are seen for smoking and drinking behaviors.

THE ROLE OF SOCIAL SUPPORT

High levels of social support can positively influence health outcomes through behavioral and psychological pathways. For example, social support may help people stick to healthier diets and reduce emotional stress. Both of these pathways can affect biological functioning in the cardiovascular, neuroendocrine, and immune systems. Social support can, therefore, both directly benefit people and indirectly buffer them from risk factors that might otherwise damage their health. In a study conducted on the relationship between psychosocial factors and atherosclerosis (plaque in the arteries), social support contributed to lower atherosclerosis levels. The protective nature of social support may be especially important for populations that experience discrimination or exclusion. One study of first-generation immigrants found that social support acted as a barrier against the harmful physical and mental health effects of discrimination.

SOCIAL ISOLATION AND ITS EFFECTS

While social ties sometimes transmit negative health behaviors or add stress, social isolation is usually detrimental to health and increases mortality. Social isolation is a special concern for older adults, as contact with friends decreases with age. Social isolation and loneliness as a result of the coronavirus 2019 (COVID-19) pandemic are likely to become major risk factors affecting the health outcomes of older adults. Another study found that younger adults in their 20s reported more social isolation than those aged 50 and older during physical distancing. Older people in long-term care facilities or with conditions that interfere with daily activities, such as arthritis, may suffer from loneliness and a lack of social cohesion, which may negatively influence health. For example, one study conducted among older adults found an association between reduced neighborhood social cohesion and a heightened likelihood of insomnia, which can have negative health effects. Similarly, during natural disasters such as heat waves, elderly people living in neighborhoods with low social cohesion may lack social support from concerned neighbors who will check on them, and they have fewer safe communal areas where they can seek refuge.

CONCLUSION

Given the complex nature of the association between social ties and health, social interventions designed to improve health vary significantly. These interventions can occur at multiple levels (e.g., family, group, neighborhood) and sometimes require cross-sector collaboration (e.g., education, public health, housing) to foster community building and improve health. Further research is needed to better understand how social cohesion affects health, as well as how it can be used to reduce health disparities. This evidence will facilitate public health efforts to address social cohesion as a social determinant of health.[1]

Section 15.2 | The Power of Social Capital in Economic Mobility

"Social capital" refers to the connections, networks, or relationships among people and the value that arises from them and can be accessed or mobilized to help individuals succeed in life. It

[1] Office of Disease Prevention and Health Promotion (ODPHP), "Social Cohesion," U.S. Department of Health and Human Services (HHS), October 6, 2020. Available online. URL: https://health.gov/healthypeople/priority-areas/social-determinants-health/literature-summaries/social-cohesion. Accessed September 25, 2024.

produces information, emotional and financial support, and other resources.

IMPORTANCE OF SOCIAL CAPITAL

Social capital can be conceptualized in multiple ways, including by the number of connections an individual has, the strength of relationships, and the nature of who is connected. Network size signals the resources an individual can potentially draw upon. However, the types of relational ties that an individual has may also matter.

- "Bonding social capital" refers to ties that exist between family members and friends within an individual's immediate network ("people like me").
- "Bridging social capital" refers to ties that exist across community members ("people different from me").

Scholars suggest that bonding social capital often results in stronger ties than bridging social capital, which is often weaker. Compared to bridging ties, low-income individuals may be able to most easily and frequently access these stronger, bonding ties to help them foster employment and self-sufficiency. However, as explained below, connections to higher-status individuals and organizations—to the extent they are available to lower-income individuals—may be able to provide more advantages and opportunities than connections to lower-status individuals and organizations.

Social capital is generally unevenly distributed throughout society. Social networks may be smaller or weaker for low-income individuals because they lack family or other social connections to institutions, such as higher education, that are critical for upward economic mobility.

SOCIAL CAPITAL FOR ECONOMIC MOBILITY

Social capital may be associated with particular types of economic outcomes. Research also suggests that the strength of social ties is important, with strong ties being more beneficial to fostering employment and self-sufficiency than weak ties.

While a large social network may be beneficial, social contacts with higher-status individuals may matter more in the search for employment opportunities.

Many low-income individuals work in flexible jobs, such as through the sharing economy, via self-employment, or during off-hours, which often create social isolation from which it may be difficult to build a strong social network.

BUILDING SOCIAL CAPITAL

The Role of Social Capital in Strengthening Relationships

Social capital building relies on creating and strengthening relationships at the individual and community levels. At the individual level, families and friends play a role in building strong ties that connect individuals to opportunities. At the community level, neighborhoods help to bring people together through both formal and informal events, strengthening both bonding and bridging social capital. Community organizations, thus, play a key role in promoting social capital by enhancing social networks. Organizations can help to foster positive relationships as a byproduct of the services they provide. In other words, if individuals are already involved with a community organization for other reasons, they will likely accrue social capital through their involvement. Organizations can also provide access to opportunities, such as providing participants with information about job openings. Local partnerships help to further enhance social networks through involvement in the local community and affiliated institutions.

Strategies for Building Trust and Relationships

Building trust and fostering a quality relationship with reciprocity require different strategies. If individuals are motivated to form relationships, activities such as one-on-one or group work at community events can help to foster the formation of social capital. Bringing community members together for a discussion of local challenges can further help to improve community-level social capital. If participants identify a shared goal for the community to accomplish during the meeting, it helps to build relationships that can exist outside the context of the meeting itself. While these strategies may seem relatively simplistic, they all share the common theme of bringing people together under shared interests to foster relationships. True social capital accrual takes time and deliberate investment in social networks.

The Role of Mentor-Mentee Relationships

Mentor-mentee relationships are also beneficial in helping to provide low-income individuals with access to job opportunities. These relationships can help youth in job training and apprenticeship programs to connect with potential mentors in their occupations of interest. Mentor-mentee relationships are of particular importance for youth who are socially isolated. Social skills are an important component of how an individual interacts in the labor market and have been associated with increased employment and higher wages. Mentor-mentee relationships can help to foster the development of social skills. Mentors can also help to transfer information about tasks required for a specific job. Furthermore, formalized mentor-mentee relationships can help to broaden individual social networks through the sharing of social capital, thereby connecting mentees to high-status individuals or institutions. Thus, these relationships can help low-income individuals to start building connections that will help them in the labor market.

Government Initiatives and Social Capital Formation

The government can play a role in social capital formation through existing federal initiatives and policies. Governmental organizations and welfare programs can connect low-income individuals to resources within the community, which may help to foster relationships. Federal initiatives designed to enhance low-income families' social networks, such as those that focus on encouraging family stability, could be improved to better target social capital formation. These programs could further emphasize the importance of connections within and outside the family for obtaining economic resources.

ENHANCING ECONOMIC MOBILITY THROUGH SOCIAL CAPITAL

Social capital can be helpful for low-income individuals in gaining access to economic mobility and employment self-sufficiency. However, social capital formation is contingent on building social networks. The number of connections, the strength of relationships, and the nature of who is connected all matter. Additional work is needed to determine how to build social capital for individuals who do not have a network or are disconnected from their social network. Future research could also clarify the benefits of social capital on economic opportunities, such as job search and wage returns. Moreover, because social capital can be defined in many ways, it is often difficult to determine conclusively the paths through which social capital contributes to employment, self-sufficiency, and mobility.

Looking forward, researchers could help programs on the ground explore a variety of ways to help low-income individuals build and leverage social capital. For example, a social capital program that is focused on economic mobility could include a peer networking component comprising engagement with peers that hold each other accountable in achieving employment goals, as well as engagement with local companies to offer job training and support outside the context of the program. This is one such strategy that may help to foster social networks that are sustained in the long run to help improve economic stability.

While many programs already exist at the local level that build or leverage social capital, few are theory-driven and have been rigorously evaluated. Future work is needed to create a strong theoretical grounding for social capital programs that focus on economic mobility and employment self-sufficiency. Furthermore, rigorous evaluations of existing programs are needed to determine their effect on building strong relationships and lasting social capital. However, despite these limitations, the potential for social capital to improve the lives and economic mobility of low-income individuals is vast.[1]

---

[1] Office of the Assistant Secretary for Planning and Evaluation (ASPE), "The Role of Social Capital in Supporting Economic Mobility," U.S. Department of Health and Human Services (HHS), May 2019. Available online. URL: https://aspe.hhs.gov/sites/default/files/private/aspe-files/261791/socialcapitalsupportingeconomicmobility.pdf. Accessed September 26, 2024.

Section 15.3 | The Health Benefits of Civic Participation

Civic participation encompasses a wide range of formal and informal activities, such as voting, volunteering, participating in group activities, and community gardening. Some are individual activities that benefit society (e.g., voting) or group activities that benefit either the group members (e.g., recreational soccer teams) or society (e.g., volunteer organizations). In addition to the direct benefit that civic participation provides to the community, it also produces secondary health benefits for participants.

BUILDING SOCIAL CAPITAL THROUGH CIVIC PARTICIPATION

One way civic participation improves health is by building social capital, which is defined as "features of social organization such as networks, norms, and social trust that facilitate coordination and cooperation for mutual benefit." For example, a study found that members of civic groups were more likely to be physically active. Belonging to civic groups expanded participants' social networks, which made them more aware of opportunities to be physically active in their community. Engaging in meaningful civic activities can also help individuals develop a sense of purpose, which may promote continued civic participation.

VOTING AND HEALTH

Participating in the electoral process by voting or registering others to vote is an example of civic participation that affects health. A study of 44 countries (including the United States) found that voter participation was associated with better self-reported health, even after controlling for individual and country characteristics. In another study, individuals who did not vote reported poorer health in subsequent years.

THE HEALTH BENEFITS OF VOLUNTEERING

Volunteering is a common form of civic participation that can yield health benefits. Studies show that volunteers enjoy better psychological well-being and more positive emotional health. Volunteering can increase social resources such as having friends to call, which may help explain the association between volunteering and reduced levels of anxiety and depressive symptoms. Additionally, one study found volunteering can relieve stress as measured by cortisol (a hormone released when feeling stressed). Volunteering might be especially beneficial for older adults; a study of adults aged 60 and older found that volunteers had a lower risk of cognitive impairment.

GROUP MEMBERSHIP AND SOCIAL ISOLATION

Simply belonging to groups can improve health as well. Membership in formal groups (e.g., Girl Scouts, Kiwanis, Rotary, PTA) or informal groups (e.g., book clubs, bird-watching clubs) has been shown to increase social capital and decrease social isolation among members. As a result, these groups may indirectly improve the physical and mental health of their members. For example, a women's group, the Red Hat Society, has been shown to provide emotional support and a sense of community to its members. Many formal and informal groups also engage in charitable activities that directly benefit health research (e.g., the Ice Bucket Challenge, Susan G. Komen Race for the Cure).

COMMUNITY GARDENING AND HEALTH

Individuals who are involved in community gardening may form a sense of neighborhood pride, experience an increased appreciation for their neighborhood, and be more motivated to get involved in community life. Community gardens also increase access to healthy foods. A thematic review of the effects of community gardens notes that 13 studies have found higher levels of fruit and vegetable consumption in areas with community gardens.

VARIATIONS IN CIVIC PARTICIPATION

Civic participation varies by generation and education. For example, one study found that while young people may be less likely to engage in mainstream media consumption, 90 percent of the high school students surveyed had engaged in politics in general and 40 percent had engaged in participatory politics. This civic engagement primarily occurs through social media. Individuals with higher education levels may have more opportunities for civic engagement, as college students have opportunities to get involved in community affairs through fraternities, sororities, or other student organizations—but male college students are less likely to engage in civic activities than female students. Other studies have found that African-American, Latino, and Asian-American college students are more likely to intend to volunteer than their white peers.

STRATEGIES TO PROMOTE CIVIC PARTICIPATION

Many strategies can promote civic participation. Encouraging young people to be active in their community is important for promoting lifelong civic participation. One study found that high school students involved in community service are more likely to vote and volunteer in adulthood. Initiatives such as AmeriCorps, which are designed to help young adults serve their communities, have been shown to increase civic participation later in life as well. Public health media advocacy campaigns are another strategy; they promote policy change through media engagement and community action.[1]

Section 15.4 | Community Engagement and Place-Based Health Interventions

Improving health is not always a matter of prescribing the right medicine. Sometimes the environment needs to change. Many Americans live in neighborhoods that lack safe walking routes, grocery stores, and health facilities.

---

[1] Office of Disease Prevention and Health Promotion (ODPHP), "Civic Participation," U.S. Department of Health and Human Services (HHS), September 23, 2020. Available online. URL: https://health.gov/healthypeople/priority-areas/social-determinants-health/literature-summaries/civic-participation. Accessed September 25, 2024.

"Are there places for kids to play? Are there good farmers markets or grocery stores?" asks Irene Dankwa-Mullan, MD, MPH, formerly of the National Institute on Minority Health and Health Disparities (NIMHD) and now deputy chief health officer of IBM Watson Health. Such features help people in a neighborhood live healthier lives. Along with NIMHD Director Eliseo Pérez-Stable, Dr. Dankwa-Mullan wrote an editorial in the April 2016 issue of the *American Journal of Public Health*, "Addressing Health Disparities Is a Place-Based Issue."

Efforts to address these problems in particular communities are called "place-based interventions." Ideally, these interventions come from a collaboration among community members, businesses, and other stakeholders, working together with police, urban planners, and other groups to improve their neighborhoods. Community members are involved to make sure the interventions are based on their values.

Examples of place-based interventions include an effort to bring a farmers market to a neighborhood without a grocery store or promoting public safety so that residents feel safe walking on the street. Walking is a simple way to improve health, but there can be many barriers to walking, a fact highlighted in the Surgeon General's *Call to Action* on walking (www.hhs.gov/surgeongeneral/reports-and-publications/physical-activity-nutrition/index.html).

Place-based interventions have been used successfully in rural areas, disadvantaged urban neighborhoods, and Indian reservations. People who live in such places tend to have particular health problems, such as diabetes and heart disease, and working to change the place-based conditions may help address health disparities.

Communities are complicated, and figuring out the best way to improve the health of all residents in a particular place can be a daunting task. "Part of the issue is that we do not have a best practices model for place-based interventions," Dr. Dankwa-Mullan says. The editorial in the *American Journal of Public Health* was part of a new series on best practices for place-based interventions. Through this series, public health professionals will be able to learn how to develop place-based interventions.

One key to the success of place-based interventions is involving the community. This is similar to community-based participatory research, a way of doing research in which the community sets priorities. This ensures that communities that are asked to participate in research get answers to the questions that are most important to them.

A research program in Baltimore is looking at bringing healthier food to African Americans who have high blood pressure (HBP) and mild or moderate chronic kidney disease. The Dietary Approaches to Stop Hypertension (DASH) diet can lower blood pressure without medication. But it can be difficult for people who live in low-income areas with few supermarkets to get the vegetables and other healthy foods that are part of the diet. In the study led by an NIMHD grantee, participants will learn about the DASH diet and receive $30 per week of potassium-rich foods. Researchers will monitor participants' blood pressure and kidney health to see whether the intervention helps.

In rural Kentucky, another NIMHD grantee is trying to improve health by teaching children about healthy foods and drinks, in cooperation with community organizations and farmers markets.

Another National Institutes of Health (NIH)-funded project in Baltimore is exploring alcohol policies that may reduce neighborhood violence. The researchers are examining how the density of liquor stores affects violence among youth.

These studies are not only delivering interventions; they are testing whether the individual interventions work to improve health. "Programs need to have evaluations or metrics of success," Dr. Dankwa-Mullan says. "We need more research on the impact." By funding research on place-based interventions, the NIMHD hopes to find out the best ways to improve the health of disadvantaged people and reduce health disparities.[1]

[1] "Working with Communities to Improve Health," National Institute on Minority Health and Health Disparities (NIMHD), May 1, 2017. Available online. URL: www.nimhd.nih.gov/news-events/features/community-health/working-with-communities.html. Accessed September 25, 2024.

Chapter 16 | **National Strategy on Gender Equity and Equality**

THE IMPORTANCE OF ADVANCING GENDER EQUITY AND EQUALITY

Advancing gender equity and equality is fundamental to every individual's economic security, safety, health, and ability to exercise their most basic rights. It is also essential to economic growth and development, democracy and political stability, and the security of nations across the globe. Ensuring that all people, regardless of gender, have the opportunity to realize their full potential is, therefore, both a moral and strategic imperative. The coronavirus 2019 (COVID-19) pandemic has fueled a health crisis, an economic crisis, and a caregiving crisis that has magnified the challenges that women and girls, especially women and girls of color, have long faced. It has also exacerbated a "shadow pandemic" of gender-based violence in the United States and around the world.

The National Strategy on Gender Equity and Equality sets forth an aspirational vision and a comprehensive agenda to advance gender equity and equality in domestic and foreign policy—and demonstrates that families, communities, and nations around the world stand to benefit.

The strategy identifies 10 interconnected priorities:

1. economic security
2. gender-based violence
3. health
4. education
5. justice and immigration

6. human rights and equality under the law
7. security and humanitarian relief
8. climate change
9. science and technology
10. democracy, participation, and leadership

The strategy also adopts an intersectional approach that considers the barriers and challenges faced by those who experience intersecting and compounding forms of discrimination and bias related to:

- gender
- race
- sexual orientation
- ethnicity
- religion
- disability
- age
- socioeconomic status

This includes addressing discrimination and bias faced by Black, Latino, Indigenous, and Native American people, Asian Americans, Native Hawaiians, Pacific Islanders, and other people of color.

STRATEGIC PRIORITIES

Improving Economic Security

- Ensure that people have equal access to good jobs by addressing persistent gender discrimination and systemic barriers to full workforce participation.
- Invest in care infrastructure and care workers to help rebuild the economy and lower costs for working families.
- Dismantle the barriers to equal opportunity in education that undermine the ability to compete on a level playing field, recognizing that education affects future economic security.

Preventing and Responding to Gender-Based Violence

- Work to eliminate gender-based violence wherever it occurs by developing and strengthening national and global laws and policies, investing in comprehensive services for survivors, and increasing prevention efforts.

- Address sexual violence in conflict settings; the elevated risk of violence facing women human rights defenders, activists, and politicians; human trafficking both at home and abroad; and the crisis of missing and murdered Indigenous people.
- Promote the safety and fair treatment of all people in the justice and immigration systems.

Increasing Access to Health Care

- Build on the historic work of the Affordable Care Act (ACA) and continue to expand and improve health care globally.
- Defend the constitutional right to safe and legal abortion in the United States, established in *Roe v. Wade*, and promote access to sexual and reproductive health and rights both at home and abroad.
- Address the pernicious effects of health inequity, including the maternal mortality crisis in the United States, which disproportionately affects Black and Native American women, and work to reduce maternal mortality and morbidity abroad.

Advancing Democracy, Rights, and Full Participation

- Work to advance gender equity and equality in the law and ensure that rights on paper are fully implemented in practice.
- Work toward gender parity and diversity in leadership roles, including in peace processes, national security and defense, global health and humanitarian efforts, and the private sector.
- Promote the leadership of women and girls in addressing the challenges of climate change and seek to close gender gaps in STEM fields so that women and girls can shape the workforce of the future.[1]

---

[1] "National Strategy on Gender Equity and Equality," The White House, October 22, 2021. Available online. URL: www.whitehouse.gov/briefing-room/statements-releases/2021/10/22/fact-sheet-national-strategy-on-gender-equity-and-equality. Accessed September 25, 2024.

Part 3 | Demographic Disparities in Health Status

Chapter 17 | **Mortality Trends across Demographic Groups**

Chapter Contents

Section 17.1 | **Mortality Trends and Life Expectancy in the United States**

The following data provide information on mortality patterns among U.S. residents by variables such as sex, age, race and Hispanic origin, and cause of death. Life expectancy estimates, age-adjusted death rates, age-specific death rates, the 10 leading causes of death, infant mortality rates, and the 10 leading causes of infant death were analyzed by comparing 2022 and 2021 final data.

HOW LONG CAN WE EXPECT TO LIVE?

In 2022, life expectancy at birth was 77.5 years for the total U.S. population—an increase of 1.1 years from 76.4 years in 2021 (see Figure 17.1). For males, life expectancy increased 1.3 years from 73.5 in 2021 to 74.8 in 2022. For females, life expectancy increased 0.9 years from 79.3 in 2021 to 80.2 in 2022.

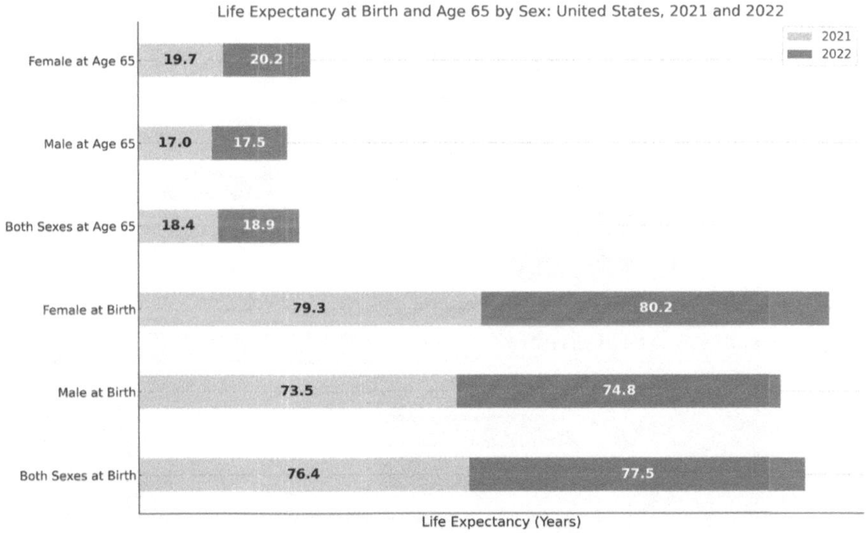

Figure 17.1. Life Expectancy at Birth and Age 65, by Sex: United States, 2021 and 2022

Centers for Disease Control and Prevention (CDC)
Source: National Center for Health Statistics, National Vital Statistics System, mortality data file.

In 2022, the difference in life expectancy between females and males was 5.4 years, a decrease of 0.4 years from 2021.

In 2022, life expectancy at age 65 for the total population was 18.9 years, an increase of 0.5 years from 2021. For males, life expectancy at age 65 increased 0.5 years from 17.0 in 2021 to 17.5 in 2022. For females, life expectancy at age 65 increased 0.5 years from 19.7 in 2021 to 20.2 in 2022. The difference in life expectancy at age 65 between females and males was 2.7 years in 2022, unchanged from 2021.

WHAT ARE THE AGE-ADJUSTED DEATH RATES FOR RACE-ETHNICITY-SEX GROUPS?

The age-adjusted death rate for the total population decreased 9.2 percent from 879.7 deaths per 100,000 U.S. standard population in 2021 to 798.8 in 2022 (see Figure 17.2).

From 2021 to 2022, age-adjusted death rates, corrected for race and ethnicity misclassification, decreased 15.4 percent for Hispanic

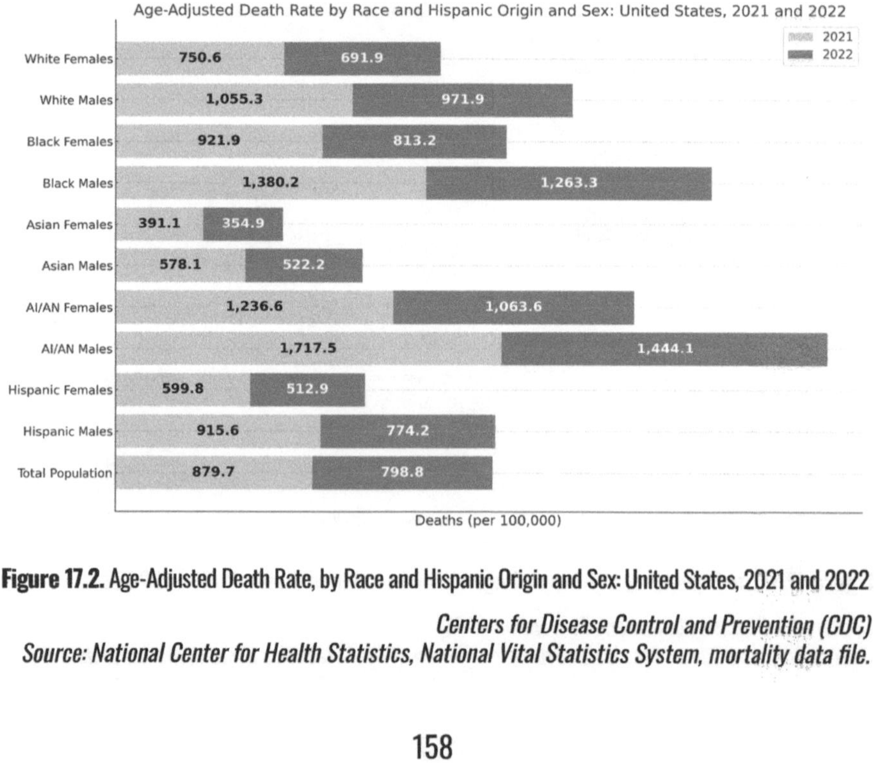

Figure 17.2. Age-Adjusted Death Rate, by Race and Hispanic Origin and Sex: United States, 2021 and 2022

Centers for Disease Control and Prevention (CDC)
Source: National Center for Health Statistics, National Vital Statistics System, mortality data file.

males (915.6 to 774.2) and 14.5 percent for Hispanic females (599.8 to 512.9). Among the non-Hispanic population, death rates decreased 15.9 percent for American Indian and Alaska Native males (1,717.5 to 1,444.1), 14.0 percent for American Indian and Alaska Native females (1,236.6 to 1,063.6), 9.7 percent for Asian males (578.1 to 522.2), 9.3 percent for Asian females (391.1 to 354.9), 8.5 percent for Black males (1,380.2 to 1,263.3), 11.8 percent for Black females (921.9 to 813.2), 7.9 percent for white males (1,055.3 to 971.9), and 7.8 percent for white females (750.6 to 691.9).

DID AGE-SPECIFIC DEATH RATES IN 2022 CHANGE FROM 2021 FOR THOSE AGE ONE YEAR AND OLDER?

From 2021 to 2022, death rates increased 12.0 percent for the age group 1–4 (from 25.0 deaths per 100,000 population in 2021 to 28.0 in 2022) and increased 7.0 percent for the age group 5–14 (14.3 to 15.3; see Figure 17.3).

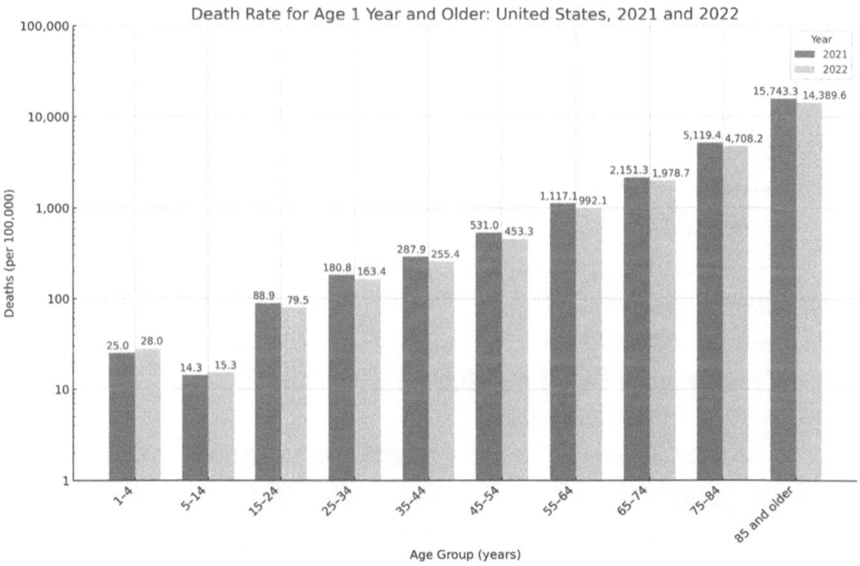

Figure 17.3. Death Rate for Age 1 Year and Older: United States, 2021 and 2022

Centers for Disease Control and Prevention (CDC)
Source: National Center for Health Statistics, National Vital Statistics System, mortality data file.

Age-specific rates decreased 10.6 percent for the age group 15–24 (88.9 to 79.5), 9.6 percent for 25–34 (180.8 to 163.4), 11.3 percent for 35–44 (287.9 to 255.4), 14.6 percent for 45–54 (531.0 to 453.3), 11.2 percent for 55–64 (1,117.1 to 992.1), 8.0 percent for 65–74 (2,151.3 to 1,978.7), 8.0 percent for 75–84 (5,119.4 to 4,708.2), and 8.6 percent for 85 and older (15,743.3 to 14,389.6).

WHAT ARE THE DEATH RATES FOR THE 10 LEADING CAUSES OF DEATH?

In 2022, the 10 leading causes of death remained the same as in 2021. The top leading cause in 2022 was heart disease, followed by cancer (see Figure 17.4).

Four causes changed rank from 2021. Unintentional injuries, the 4th leading cause of death in 2021, became the 3rd leading cause in 2022, while coronavirus 2019 (COVID-19) dropped from the 3rd leading cause to the fourth. Kidney disease went from the 10th leading cause in 2021 to the 9th leading cause in 2022, while

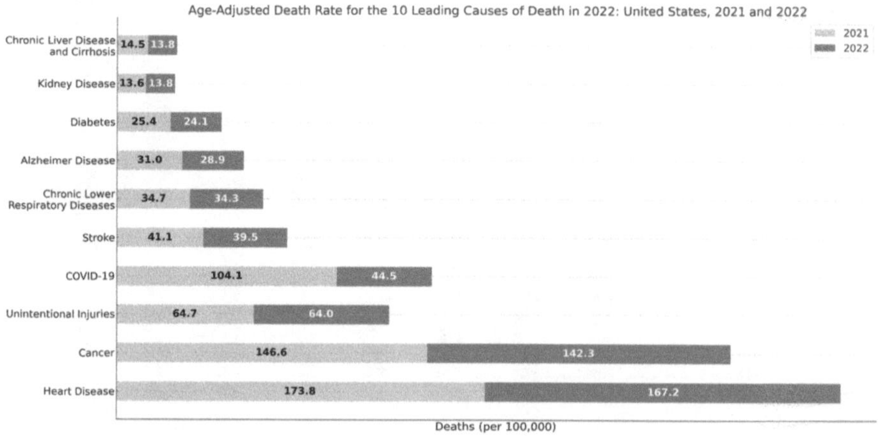

Figure 17.4. Age-Adjusted Death Rate for the 10 Leading Causes of Death in 2022: United States, 2021 and 2022

Centers for Disease Control and Prevention (CDC)
Source: National Center for Health Statistics, National Vital Statistics System, mortality data file.

chronic liver disease and cirrhosis dropped from the 9th leading cause to the 10th. The remaining leading causes in 2022 (stroke, chronic lower respiratory diseases, Alzheimer disease, and diabetes) remained at the same ranks as in 2021.

From 2021 to 2022, age-adjusted death rates decreased for 9 of the 10 leading causes of death and increased for one. The rate decreased 3.8 percent for heart disease (from 173.8 in 2021 to 167.2 in 2022), 2.9 percent for cancer (146.6 to 142.3), 1.1 percent for unintentional injuries (64.7 to 64.0), 57.3 percent for COVID-19 (104.1 to 44.5), 3.9 percent for stroke (41.1 to 39.5), 1.2 percent for chronic lower respiratory diseases (34.7 to 34.3), 6.8 percent for Alzheimer disease (AD; 31.0 to 28.9), 5.1 percent for diabetes (25.4 to 24.1), and 4.8 percent for chronic liver disease and cirrhosis (14.5 to 13.8).

The rate increased 1.5 percent for kidney disease (13.6 to 13.8).

WHAT ARE THE MORTALITY RATES FOR THE 10 LEADING CAUSES OF INFANT DEATH AND FOR INFANT DEATHS OVERALL?

The infant mortality rate (IMR) increased 3.1 percent from 543.6 infant deaths per 100,000 live births in 2021 to 560.4 in 2022.

Causes of infant death are ranked according to the number of infant deaths. The 10 leading causes of infant death in 2022 (congenital malformations, low birth weight, sudden infant death syndrome, unintentional injuries, maternal complications, cord and placental complications, bacterial sepsis of newborn, respiratory distress of newborn, intrauterine hypoxia and birth asphyxia, and diseases of the circulatory system) accounted for 65.2 percent of all infant deaths in the United States (see Figure 17.5).

In 2022, intrauterine hypoxia and birth asphyxia moved from the 10th leading cause of infant death to the 9th leading cause, while diseases of the circulatory system dropped from the 9th to the 10th leading cause. The IMR for maternal complications increased 8.9 percent from 30.4 in 2021 to 33.1 in 2022, and the IMR for bacterial sepsis of newborn increased 13.8 percent (15.2 to 17.3).

Mortality rates for the other leading causes of infant death did not change significantly.

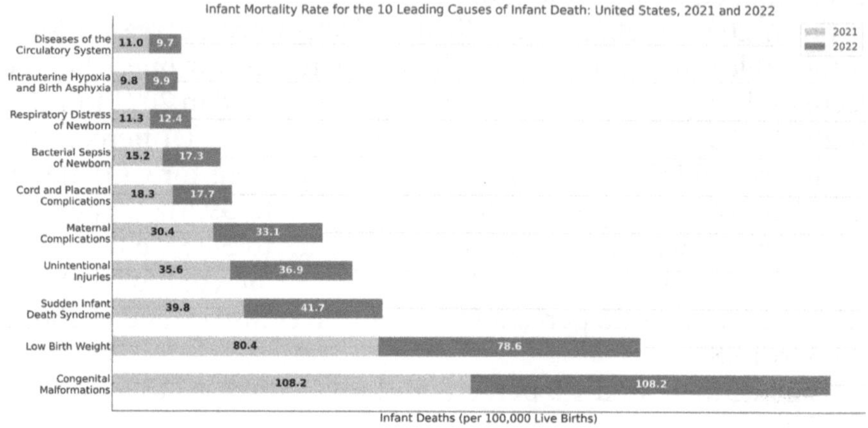

Figure 17.5. Infant Mortality Rate for the 10 Leading Causes of Infant Death in 2022: United States, 2021 and 2022

Centers for Disease Control and Prevention (CDC)
Source: National Center for Health Statistics, National Vital Statistics System, mortality data file.

SUMMARY

In 2022, a total of 3,279,857 resident deaths were registered in the United States—184,374 fewer deaths than in 2021. The number of deaths for which COVID-19 was the underlying cause of death decreased 55.3 percent from 416,893 in 2021 to 186,552 in 2022. COVID-19 dropped from the third leading cause to the fourth. The age-adjusted death rate for the total population decreased 9.2 percent in 2022 from 2021 after an increase of 5.3 percent from 2020 to 2021. Life expectancy for the total population increased 1.1 years from 2021 to 2022. Age-specific death rates from 2021 to 2022 increased for age groups 1–4 and 5–14 and decreased for each age group 15–24 years and older. Age-adjusted death rates decreased in 2022 from 2021 for all race and Hispanic-origin groups for both males and females.

The 10 leading causes of death in 2022 remained the same as in 2021. Heart disease was the leading cause of death, followed by cancer. Age-adjusted death rates decreased for nine leading causes and increased for one. Life expectancy at birth increased 1.1 years from 76.4 in 2021 to 77.5 in 2022, largely because of decreases in mortality due to COVID-19, heart disease, cancer, unintentional injuries, and homicide.

In 2022, 20,553 deaths occurred in children younger than 1 year, which was 633 more infant deaths than in 2021. The IMR increased 3.1 percent from 543.6 infant deaths per 100,000 live births in 2021 to 560.4 in 2022. Among the 10 leading causes of infant death, the increase in IMR for two causes (maternal complications and bacterial sepsis of newborn) was significant.[1]

Section 17.2 | Mortality due to Firearm Injury and Death

FIREARM INJURY AND DEATH

A firearm injury is a wound or penetrating injury from a weapon that uses a powder charge to fire a projectile. Weapons that use a powder charge include handguns, rifles, and shotguns. Injuries from air- and gas-powered guns, BB guns, and pellet guns are not considered firearm injuries. This is because these types of guns do not use a powder charge to fire a projectile.

Firearm injuries and deaths continue to be a significant public health problem in the United States. While firearm violence and injury affect people in all communities, some groups have higher rates of firearm injury than others. In 2022, there were more than 48,000 firearm-related deaths in the United States according to mortality data. That is about 132 people dying from a firearm-related injury each day. More than half of firearm-related deaths were suicides, and more than 4 out of every 10 were firearm homicides.

More people suffer nonfatal firearm-related injuries than die. More than 7 out of every 10 medically treated firearm injuries are from firearm-related assaults. Nearly 2 out of every 10 are from unintentional firearm injuries. There are few intentionally self-inflicted

[1] "Mortality in the United States, 2022," Centers for Disease Control and Prevention (CDC), March 2024. Available online. URL: www.cdc.gov/nchs/data/databriefs/db492.pdf. Accessed September 26, 2024.

firearm-related injuries seen in hospital emergency departments. Most people who use a firearm in a suicide attempt die from their injury.

Firearm injuries affect people in all stages of life. In 2022, firearm injuries (all types) were among the five leading causes of death for people aged 1–44 in the United States. Firearm injuries were the leading cause of death among children and teens aged 1–19.

WHO IS AFFECTED?

Some groups have higher rates of firearm injury than others. Men account for 86 percent of all victims of firearm death and 87 percent of firearm injuries.

Rates of firearm violence vary by age, race, and ethnicity. Firearm homicide rates are highest among:

- teens and young adults aged 15–34
- Black or African-American individuals
- American Indian or Alaska Native individuals
- Hispanic or Latino individuals

Firearm suicide rates are highest among:

- adults aged 75 and older
- American Indian or Alaska Native individuals
- non-Hispanic white individuals

These inequities underscore the importance of addressing the social and structural conditions that drive rates of violence and suicide.

CONSEQUENCES

People who survive a firearm-related injury may experience long-term consequences. These include problems with memory, thinking, emotions, physical disability from injury to the brain, and paralysis from spinal cord injuries. Chronic mental health problems from conditions such as posttraumatic stress disorder (PTSD) are also included.

The effects of firearm violence and injury extend beyond victims and their families. Shooting incidents, including those in homes, schools, houses of worship, workplaces, shopping areas, on the street, or at community events, can affect the sense of safety and security of entire communities and affect everyday decisions.

The economic consequence of firearm violence is also substantial. Firearm violence and injury cost the United States tens of billions of dollars each year in medical and lost productivity costs.

PREVENTION

Firearm injuries and deaths are preventable—not inevitable—and everyone has a role to play in prevention. A comprehensive approach and partnerships working with communities can reduce inequities and prevent firearm deaths and injuries.[1]

Section 17.3 | COVID-19 Mortality Disparities across Race, Ethnicity, and Gender

Males and the Hispanic, American Indian, and Alaska Native (AIAN) populations experienced a disproportionately large number of deaths from 2019 to 2020, the year that included the start of the coronavirus 2019 (COVID-19) pandemic.

Deaths for the total U.S. population increased 19 percent in 2020, but some groups were more affected than others, according to the U.S. Census Bureau's Vintage 2022 Population Estimates released today—the first to contain final 2020 mortality data by demographic characteristics.

There were large increases in deaths across all demographic groups between 2019 and 2020 and smaller increases for most groups from 2020 to 2021. Deaths declined for all groups from 2021 to 2022.

[1] "Fast Facts: Firearm Injury and Death," Centers for Disease Control and Prevention (CDC), July 5, 2024. Available online. URL: www.cdc.gov/firearm-violence/data-research/facts-stats/index.html. Accessed September 30, 2024.

Increases in deaths during 2020 were reflected in previous estimates releases, but the latest data show the disproportionate effect of the pandemic on mortality by race, ethnicity, and sex.

MORTALITY TRENDS BY CHARACTERISTICS

There were large increases in deaths across all demographic groups between 2019 and 2020, and smaller increases for most groups from 2020 to 2021 (see Table 17.1). Deaths declined for all groups from 2021 to 2022.

MORTALITY BY SEX

Males have historically had higher death rates than females, and for most of the last decade, the gap between the two sexes had been growing prior to the pandemic. In 2012, for example, 50.1 percent of deaths were male. By 2019, the share had increased to 51.6 percent.

Between 2019 and 2020, male deaths increased by 296,061 (20.1%) and female deaths by 232,830 (16.9%). The trend continued in 2021, with 68,208 (3.9%) more male deaths and 12,298 (0.8%) more female deaths.

In 2021, 53.1 percent of those who died were male. Provisional 2022 National Center for Health Statistics (NCHS) data show larger declines for males, but the share of male deaths (52.4%) was still larger than in pre-pandemic years.

The growing difference in deaths between males and females in 2020 and 2021 suggests the COVID-19 pandemic had a larger effect on the mortality of males than it did on females.

HISPANIC ORIGIN

Because the Hispanic population comprises a much smaller share of the total population relative to the non-Hispanic group, the majority of deaths are non-Hispanic.

Similarly, as the share of the Hispanic population increased from 2010 to 2020, so did the share of deaths among this group, which went from 6.2 percent in 2012 to 7 percent in 2017 and 7.4 percent in 2019.

Table 17.1. Estimates of U.S. Deaths and Annual Change by Sex, Hispanic Origin and Race: 2019–2022

	Deaths				Annual Numeric Change				Annual Percent Change			
Characteristic	**2019**	**2020**	**2021**	**2022**	**2019**	**2020**	**2021**	**2022**	**2019**	**2020**	**2021**	**2022**
Sex												
Female	1,381,015	1,613,845	1,626,123	1,558,144	279	232,830	12,298	–67,979	0.02	16.86	0.76	–4.18
Male	1,473,823	1,769,884	1,838,108	1,715,561	15,354	296,061	68,208	–122,547	1.05	20.09	3.85	–6.67
Hispanic Origin												
Non-Hispanic	2,642,441	3,078,021	3,148,567	2,998,451	7,955	435,580	70,546	–150,116	0.30	16.48	2.29	–4.77
Hispanic	212,397	305,708	315,664	275,254	7,678	93,311	9,956	–40,410	3.75	43.93	3.26	–12.80
One Race												
White	2,393,548	2,785,557	2,859,254	2,716,557	7,509	392,009	73,697	–142,697	0.31	16.38	2.65	–4.99
Black or African American	351,907	465,491	456,419	417,232	5,374	104,584	–72	–39,187	1.55	29.72	–0.02	–8.59
Alaska Native	19,227	26,276	28,941	25,216	380	7,049	2,665	–3,725	2.02	36.66	10.14	–12.87
Asian	71,420	92,439	93,763	90,298	1,731	21,019	1,324	–3,465	2.48	29.43	1.43	–3.70
Native Hawaiian and other Pacific Islander	3,805	4,865	5,636	4,994	266	1,060	771	–642	7.52	27.86	15.85	–11.39
Two or more races	14,931	18,101	20,218	19,408	373	3,170	2,117	–810	2.56	21.23	11.70	–4.01

Source: U.S. Census Bureau, Vintage 2022 National Population Estimates.

The increase in Hispanic deaths between 2019 and 2020, however, represents a notable break in the time series, jumping from 7.4 to 9 percent of all deaths in a single year. The Hispanic population's share of mortality increased again (9.1%) in 2021, the first full year of the pandemic.

The increase in Hispanic mortality during the pandemic was higher relative to the non-Hispanic U.S. population, though it declined slightly to 8.4 percent of total deaths in 2022, according to provisional data.

RACE GROUPS

All race groups experienced higher-than-normal increases in deaths from 2019 to 2020. However, during the pandemic's first year, every race group other than the white population experienced single-year percentage increases higher than the 18.5 percent increase in deaths for the total population.

Prior to the pandemic, mortality increases in the previous decade were relatively small and did not vary significantly annually across races.

The following trends in mortality rates are noteworthy:

- In 2020, the largest mortality increase occurred in the American Indian and Alaska Native population (36.7%), followed by the Black (29.7%) and Asian (29.4%) populations.
- In 2021, there was more variation in the magnitude and direction of change across groups. Black deaths decreased by less than 1 percent between 2020 and 2021, while the Native Hawaiian and Other Pacific Islander (15.9%), Two or More Races (11.7%), and American Indian and Alaska Native (10.1%) populations continued to experience larger percentage increases in deaths than the total population.
- White deaths (2.65%) were also slightly higher than the total increase (2.38%).
- Provisional 2022 data show declines in mortality for all race groups between 2021 and 2022, with

the largest declines occurring among the American Indian and Alaska Native (−12.9%) and Native Hawaiian and Other Pacific-Islander (−11.4%) populations.[1]

[1] "COVID-19 Impacts on Mortality by Race/Ethnicity and Sex," United States Census Bureau, June 22, 2023. Available online. URL: www.census.gov/library/stories/2023/06/covid-19-impacts-on-mortality-by-race-ethnicity-and-sex.html. Accessed September 27, 2024.

Chapter 18 | Barriers to Health-Care Access and Utilization

Chapter Contents

Section 18.1 | **Health-Care Coverage and Expenditures in the United States**

In 2022, the United States had an estimated population of 328 million people. Most of those individuals had private health insurance or were covered under a federal program (such as Medicare or Medicaid). About 8 percent of the U.S. population was uninsured. Individuals (including those who were uninsured), health insurers, and federal and state governments spent approximately $4.2 trillion on various types of health consumption expenditures (HCE) in 2022, which accounted for 16.5 percent of the nation's gross domestic product.

Table 18.1 presents data on health-care coverage in the United States for 2022, showing the enrollment figures and percentages of the population covered by various types of insurance.

Table 18.1. Health-Care Coverage, 2022

Source	**Enrollment (Millions/Percentage of U.S. Population)**
Insured	302 (92%)
Private Health Insurance—Group	180 (54.8%)
Private Health Insurance—Direct-Purchase	46 (13.9%)
Medicaid/CHIP	70 (21.2%)
Medicare	61 (18.5%)
Military—TRICARE	9 (2.7%)
Military—VA Care	7 (2.2%)
Uninsured	26 (8%)

Source: U.S. Census Bureau, American Community Survey, September 2023.

PRIVATE HEALTH INSURANCE

Private health insurance is the predominant source of health insurance coverage in the United States. It includes both group coverage (largely made up of employer-sponsored insurance) and direct-purchase coverage (which includes plans directly purchased from an insurer both on the health insurance exchanges and outside of them). In 2022, an estimated 180 million individuals (54.8% of the U.S. population) were covered by group coverage, and 46 million individuals (13.9% of the U.S. population) were covered by direct-purchase coverage.

In 2022, private health insurance expenditures accounted for $1,290 billion (30.4% of overall HCE). Private health insurance expenditures include amounts paid by insuring organizations to providers and all insuring organizations' nonmedical net costs, which include but are not limited to taxes, net gains or losses to reserves, and profits. A majority of this spending was for hospital care and physician and professional services. Private health insurance spending experienced a decline from 2019 to 2020, predominantly caused by enrollment decreases and lower health-care utilization stemming from the coronavirus 2019 (COVID-19) pandemic, but it has since rebounded.

MEDICARE

Medicare is a federal health insurance program that pays for covered health-care services for most people aged 65 and older and for certain permanently disabled individuals under the age of 65.

An estimated 61 million individuals (18.5% of the U.S. population) were enrolled in Medicare in 2022. The program accounted for $944 billion (22.2% of overall HCE); this share is about 10 percentage points higher than Medicare's percentage of HCE in 1970. In 2022, most of the spending was for hospital care and physician and professional services.

MEDICAID/CHIP

Medicaid is a joint federal-state program that finances the delivery of primary and acute medical services, as well as long-term services and supports, to a diverse low-income population, including children, pregnant women, adults, individuals with disabilities, and people aged 65 and older. The State Children's Health Insurance

Program (CHIP) is a means-tested program that provides health coverage to targeted low-income children and pregnant women in families with annual incomes above Medicaid eligibility levels but no health insurance.

An estimated 70 million individuals (21.2% of the U.S. population) received Medicaid or CHIP in 2022, and the programs accounted for $829 billion (19.5% of overall HCE). This spending is about 12 percentage points higher than Medicaid/CHIP's percentage of total HCE in 1970. Furthermore, relative to other coverage, Medicaid spends the highest percentage of its expenditures on long-term services and supports, which include:

- other health, residential, and personal care
- nursing care facilities and continuing care retirement communities
- home health care

MILITARY

The U.S. Department of Defense (DOD) provides health-care services for military service members, veterans, and their dependents through programs such as TRICARE and the U.S. Department of Veterans Affairs (VA). In 2022, an estimated 9 million individuals (2.7% of the U.S. population) had TRICARE, and 7 million (2.2% of the U.S. population) had VA care. Together, these departments accounted for $148 billion (3.5% of total HCE).

OTHER HEALTH SERVICES

Other health-care spending covers services provided through public and private programs not listed above, including worksite health-care programs, philanthropic support, Indian Health Service activities, workers' compensation, general assistance, the Maternal and Child Health program, vocational rehabilitation, Substance Abuse and Mental Health Services Administration (SAMHSA) grants, federal and state public health activities, school health programs, and other programs whose primary focus is the provision of care or treatment of disease. Other health services saw a sharp, temporary increase in spending in 2020 to $752 billion (19% of total

HCE). This increase was primarily due to federal health spending addressing the COVID-19 pandemic, such as Paycheck Protection Program loans, Provider Relief Fund payments, and public health activities. Federal spending addressing COVID-19 continued to decline in 2022, contributing to the decline in other health-care spending to $564 billion (13.3% of total HCE).

OUT-OF-POCKET SPENDING

Out-of-pocket spending (other than premiums) includes all amounts paid by the privately insured and other insured individuals for coinsurance, deductibles, and services not covered by insurance. It also includes amounts paid by the uninsured for health-care goods and services. Among all individuals, out-of-pocket spending was $471 billion (11.1% of total HCE) in 2022, with roughly 30 percent attributable to durable medical equipment and other nondurable medical products.

THE UNINSURED

Approximately, 26 million individuals (8% of the U.S. population) were uninsured in 2022. Historically, the uninsured rate was relatively stable from 2008 to 2013 before dropping 6 percent points by 2016 to 8.6 percent. This drop in the uninsured rate corresponds with increases in direct-purchase and Medicaid/CHIP coverage, which are associated with the implementation of various provisions of the Patient Protection and Affordable Care Act (ACA; P.L. 111-148, as amended), such as the exchanges, premium tax credit, and Medicaid expansion. Since 2016, the uninsured rate slowly increased to 9.2 percent in 2019 before falling to 8 percent in 2022. This decline corresponds with increases in direct-purchase and Medicaid/CHIP coverage, which were affected by policies enacted in response to the COVID-19 pandemic.

The cost of care for the uninsured population is accounted for in multiple spending categories. Payments made by uninsured individuals for health-care services are included in the out-of-pocket total. Any amounts received by providers that help to partially and/or indirectly cover the cost of care for the uninsured are accounted for in corresponding source totals (e.g., Medicare and Medicaid disproportionate share hospital payments are included in program totals).[1]

Section 18.2 | Access to Affordable Medicines and Treatments

The U.S. Department of Health and Human Services (HHS), through the Centers for Medicare & Medicaid Services (CMS), finalized a rule in April 2023 to prioritize people with Medicare and implement strong protections to ensure that Medicare Advantage (MA) works effectively for them. This final rule aims to strengthen Medicare Advantage and hold health insurance companies to higher standards for America's seniors and people with disabilities. Key provisions include cracking down on misleading marketing schemes by Medicare Advantage plans, Part D plans, and their downstream entities; removing barriers to care created by complex coverage criteria and utilization management; and expanding access to behavioral health care. The new rule will also promote health equity and implement a key provision of the Inflation Reduction Act, improving access to affordable prescription drug coverage for an estimated 300,000 low-income individuals.

CRACKING DOWN ON MISLEADING MARKETING SCHEMES

The final rule includes changes to protect individuals exploring Medicare Advantage and Part D coverage from confusing and potentially misleading marketing practices. Advertisements will be prohibited if they do not mention a specific plan name or if they use the Medicare name, CMS logo, and products or information

[1] "U.S. Health-Care Coverage and Spending," Congressional Research Service (CRS), March 20, 2024. Available online. URL: https://crsreports.congress.gov/product/pdf/IF/IF10830. Accessed September 30, 2024.

issued by the federal government, including the Medicare card, in a misleading way. Furthermore, the final rule strengthens accountability for plans to monitor agent and broker activity.

REMOVING BARRIERS TO CARE CREATED BY COMPLEX PRIOR AUTHORIZATION AND UTILIZATION MANAGEMENT

The CMS is also providing important protections regarding utilization management policies and coverage criteria to ensure that Medicare Advantage enrollees receive the same access to medically necessary care as they would in Traditional Medicare. The rule streamlines prior authorization requirements and reduces disruptions for enrollees by requiring that a granted prior authorization approval remains valid for as long as medically necessary. Additionally, it mandates that Medicare Advantage plans annually review utilization management policies and that denials of coverage based on medical necessity be reviewed by health-care professionals with relevant expertise before a denial can be issued. These policies complement proposals in the CMS's Advancing Interoperability and Improving Prior Authorization Processes Proposed Rule (CMS-0057-P).

EXPANDING ACCESS TO BEHAVIORAL HEALTH CARE

The CMS remains committed to emphasizing the critical role that access to behavioral health plays in whole-person care. In line with the CMS's Behavioral Health Strategy and the administration's strategy to address the national mental health crisis, the CMS is strengthening behavioral health network adequacy in Medicare Advantage by adding clinical psychologists and licensed clinical social workers to the list of evaluated specialties. The CMS is also finalizing wait time standards for behavioral health and primary care services, along with more specific notice requirements from plans to patients when these providers are dropped from their networks. Additionally, the CMS is requiring most types of Medicare Advantage plans to include behavioral health services in care coordination programs, ensuring that behavioral health care is a core part of person-centered care planning.

PROMOTING MORE EQUITABLE CARE

Furthermore, the CMS is advancing health equity and driving quality in health coverage by establishing a health equity index in the Star Ratings program that will reward Medicare Advantage and Medicare Part D plans that provide excellent care for underserved populations. Plans will also be required to provide culturally competent care to an expanded list of populations and to improve equitable access to care for those with limited English proficiency through newly expanded requirements for providing materials in alternate formats and languages. The final rule balances patient experience and complaints measures, access measures, and health outcomes measures in the Star Ratings program to more effectively focus on patient-centric care and improving clinical outcomes.[1]

Section 18.3 | Addressing Language Barriers in Health Care

LANGUAGE ACCESS FOR INDIVIDUALS WITH LIMITED ENGLISH PROFICIENCY

Language barriers experienced by people with limited English proficiency (LEP) can lead to disparities in health-care access and health outcomes. To demonstrate its commitment to promoting meaningful language access and mitigating gaps in care, the U.S. Department of Health and Human Services's (HHS) Office of Minority Health (OMH) is joining agencies across the federal government in the release of a 2024–2026 Language Access Plan (LAP; https://minorityhealth.hhs.gov/language-access). The OMH LAP is available in nine languages.

The release of the OMH LAP coincides with the 24th anniversary of the signing of Executive Order (EO) 13166, "Improving

[1] "HHS Finalizes Rule to Strengthen Medicare, Improve Access to Affordable Prescription Drug Coverage, and Hold Private Insurance Companies Accountable to Delivering Quality Health Care for America's Seniors and People with Disabilities," U.S. Department of Health and Human Services (HHS), April 5, 2023. Available online. URL: www.hhs.gov/about/news/2023/04/05/hhs-finalizes-rule-strengthen-medicare-improve-access-affordable-prescription-drug-coverage-hold-private-insurance-companies-accountable.html. Accessed September 30, 2024.

Access to Services for Persons with Limited English Proficiency." EO 13166 requires that all federal agencies improve access to federal programs and activities for individuals with LEP.

KEY FOCUS AREAS OF THE OMH LANGUAGE ACCESS PLAN

The OMH LAP outlines five areas in which the OMH will promote meaningful language access and engagement for individuals and organizations that use its resources:

Enhancing Awareness and Promotion of the National Standards for Culturally and Linguistically Appropriate Services (CLAS) in Health and Health Care

The National CLAS Standards consist of 15 action steps that provide a blueprint for individuals and health organizations to eliminate health disparities and promote equity. The OMH encourages the adoption of the National CLAS Standards in its grant initiatives and by providing free, accredited e-learning programs and other resources through Think Cultural Health (https://thinkculturalhealth.hhs.gov/education).

Increasing Use of Translation and Interpretation Services

The OMH aims to enhance the availability and use of translation and interpretation services to improve communication and care for individuals with LEP.

Improving Language Accessibility to OMH Resources and Convenings

Efforts will be made to ensure that OMH resources and events are accessible to individuals with LEP, promoting broader participation and engagement.

Researching, Developing, and Testing Methods of Informing Individuals with LEP about the Availability of Language Assistance Services

Congress called upon the OMH in the FY 2023 budget to research, develop, and test methods of informing individuals with LEP that health-care language assistance services are available. The OMH was asked to establish a universal symbol that signals language assistance services offered in health settings. To date, the OMH has conducted research, held multiple listening sessions, and published a Request for Information (www.federalregister.gov/documents/2024/04/19/2024-08409/development-of-a-universal-symbol-for-language-assistance-services-in-health-settings) in April 2024 soliciting input from partners to inform the development of this universal symbol. The OMH will continue working with vested parties to ensure community engagement for user testing and any refinement of the symbol.

Continuing OMH Engagement in HHS Language Access Efforts

This includes serving on the HHS Language Access Steering Committee to further the objectives of improving language access across federal health programs.

Additional Initiatives

IMPROVING ACCESS TO HEALTH HAZARD EVALUATIONS

The OMH worked in partnership with the Centers for Disease Control and Prevention and the National Institute for Occupational Safety and Health to expand access to the Health Hazard Evaluation request form (www.cdc.gov/niosh/hhe/request.html)—previously available only in English and Spanish—by adding versions translated in Mixtecan, Arabic, Chinese, Vietnamese, Tagalog, and Haitian Creole. The release of the translated forms correlated with Farmworker Appreciation Day and aligns with the HHS Secretary's Initiative on Protecting Farmworkers from Extreme Heat and Wildfire Smoke. Workers can now request the form in any of the newly added languages.

ADVANCING EQUITY FOR ASIAN-AMERICAN, NATIVE HAWAIIAN, AND PACIFIC-ISLANDER COMMUNITIES IN COVID-19 RESPONSE EFFORTS

The OMH developed a set of resource guides to provide guidance on best practices to advance cultural competency, language access, and sensitivity toward Asian-American, Native Hawaiian, and Pacific-Islander communities in the federal coronavirus 2019 (COVID-19) response. The set includes an introductory document and three resource guides in English and multiple Asian, Native Hawaiian, and Pacific-Islander languages. The guides align with the Presidential Memorandum Condemning and Combating Racism, Xenophobia, and Intolerance Against Asian Americans and Pacific Islanders in the United States.

PROMOTING EQUITABLE ACCESS TO LANGUAGE SERVICES

In October 2022, the OMH announced more than $4 million in grants for the Promoting Equitable Access to Language Services (PEALS) in Health and Human Services initiative. Through the PEALS initiative, grant recipients are evaluating strategies to enhance language assistance services, including policy development and implementation, technology use, education for individuals with LEP, and education for providers, including medical support staff.

For more detailed information about how OMH is supporting language access, visit the LAP web page (https://minorityhealth.hhs.gov/language-access).[1]

Section 18.4 | Health-Care Disparities in Rural America

HEALTH-CARE ACCESS IN RURAL AREAS

More than 60 million Americans—about one-fifth of the U.S. population—live in rural areas. On average, rural residents are older and generally have worse health conditions than urban residents. However, while they may require more medical attention and care, they often face more limited access to health care.

[1] Office of Minority Health (OMH), "Language Access: A Source for Better Health," U.S. Department of Health and Human Services (HHS), August 5, 2024. Available online. URL: https://minorityhealth.hhs.gov/news/language-access-source-better-health. Accessed September 30, 2024.

HOSPITAL CLOSURES AND HIGHER RISKS

Having a local hospital or access to care is critical in emergency situations where minutes can make a significant difference. Many rural residents are experiencing the closure of their local hospitals. More than 100 rural hospitals (or 4% of all rural hospitals) closed from 2013 through 2020. As a result, residents have had to travel about 20 miles farther for common services, such as inpatient care, and 40 miles farther for less common services, such as alcohol or drug misuse treatment.

Additionally, rural areas without hospitals generally have fewer health-care providers compared to those that have not experienced closures. Consequently, people in rural areas must travel farther to access health-care services after the closure of local hospitals.

In addition to losing access to hospitals, rural residents may face additional health risks. Often, rural residents lack insurance coverage, which is associated with reduced access to care and increased risk of poor health outcomes. Many rural residents may turn to telehealth services—health care delivered via phone or video—when local care is unavailable. While telehealth can help address limited provider availability in rural areas, as of 2019, at least 17 percent of people living in rural areas lacked broadband Internet access, compared to only 1 percent of people in urban areas.

CERTAIN POPULATIONS ARE DISPROPORTIONATELY AFFECTED

While rural communities face access and quality of care challenges, some populations encounter unique difficulties. Pregnant individuals, American Indians and Alaska Natives, and veterans may struggle to access necessary care in rural areas.

For example, more than half of rural counties lacked hospital-based obstetric services in 2018. By 2030, the anticipated supply of obstetricians and gynecologists (OB/GYNs) is expected to meet only about 50 percent of the demand in rural areas. The loss of hospital-based obstetric care in rural counties is associated with increases in preterm births, and longer distances traveled for obstetric care, which may contribute to poor maternal and adverse infant health outcomes. These negative outcomes have been more prevalent in rural areas and among non-white racial and ethnic groups, particularly for Black and American Indian or Alaska Native populations.

About one-third of veterans enrolled in the Veterans Health Administration (VHA) live in rural areas. However, a review of VHA data found that rural veterans utilize intensive mental health-care services, such as residential care or intensive case management, less than their urban counterparts, raising questions about access.

The VHA's Office of Rural Health is dedicated to improving the health and well-being of rural veterans. In FY 2022, the office allocated approximately $245 million for 35 separate initiatives, including transportation for veterans to VA facilities. However, the office does not effectively communicate all of its funding opportunities across the VA. As a result, the VHA may miss opportunities to fund research at VA facilities serving rural veterans with unique access issues.

WHAT SHOULD THE FEDERAL GOVERNMENT DO?

Numerous federal agencies are involved in ensuring that rural communities have access to health care. However, more action is needed by these entities. Important recommendations have been made to improve the information available to federal agencies and help them understand and address the health-care needs of rural populations. Considering the health-care challenges faced by rural populations and the availability of financial incentives is crucial when developing programs for these communities. For more information about these recommendations and policy options, refer to the new Health Care Capsule (www.gao.gov/products/gao-23-106651).[1]

[1] "Why Health Care Is Harder to Access in Rural America," U.S. Government Accountability Office (GAO), May 16, 2023. Available online. URL: www.gao.gov/blog/why-health-care-harder-access-rural-america. Accessed September 30, 2024.

Chapter 19 | Health and Economic Costs of Chronic Conditions

Chronic diseases account for most illnesses, disability, and death in the United States and are the leading drivers of health-care costs. Ninety percent of the nation's $4.5 trillion in annual health-care expenditures are for people with chronic and mental health conditions. Interventions to prevent and manage these diseases can have significant health and economic benefits.

DISEASES

Heart Disease and Stroke

Nothing kills more Americans than heart disease and stroke. More than 944,800 Americans die of heart disease or stroke every year—that is more than one in three deaths. These diseases take an economic toll as well, costing our health-care system $254 billion per year and causing $168 billion in lost productivity on the job. Costs from cardiovascular diseases are projected to hit roughly $2 trillion by 2050.

Cancer

Each year in the United States, 1.7 million people are diagnosed with cancer, and more than 600,000 die from it, making it the second leading cause of death. The cost of cancer care continues to rise and is expected to reach more than $240 billion by 2030.

Diabetes

More than 38 million Americans have diabetes, and another 98 million adults in the United States have prediabetes, which puts them at risk for type 2 diabetes. Diabetes can cause serious complications, including heart disease, kidney failure, and blindness. In 2022, the total estimated cost of diagnosed diabetes was $413 billion in medical costs and lost productivity.

Obesity

Obesity affects 20 percent of children and 42 percent of adults, putting them at risk of chronic diseases such as type 2 diabetes, heart disease, and some cancers. Just over one in three young adults aged 17–24 are too heavy to join the U.S. military. Obesity costs the U.S. health-care system nearly $173 billion a year.

Arthritis

Arthritis affects 53.2 million adults in the United States, which is about one in five adults. It is a leading cause of disability in the United States and a leading cause of chronic pain. Arthritis-attributable medical costs and earning losses were over $300 billion in 2013.

Alzheimer Disease

Alzheimer disease (AD), a type of dementia, is an irreversible, progressive brain disease that affects nearly 7 million Americans, including one in nine adults aged 65 and older. Two-thirds of these older adults (4.2 million) are women. Deaths due to Alzheimer's disease more than doubled between 2000 and 2021, increasing 141 percent. The cost of caring for people with Alzheimer's and other dementias is an estimated $360 billion in 2024, with projected increases to nearly $1 trillion (in today's dollars) by 2050.

Epilepsy

In the United States, about 3 million adults and about half a million children and teens younger than 18 have active epilepsy—meaning that they have been diagnosed by a doctor, are taking epilepsy medicines, had a recent seizure, or both. Adults with epilepsy report worse physical and mental health and more work limitations compared to adults without epilepsy. In 2019, total health-care costs (epilepsy-attributable and other health-related costs) for noninstitutionalized people with epilepsy were $13.4 billion, of which $5.4 billion were directly attributable to epilepsy.

Tooth Decay

Cavities (also called "tooth decay") are one of the most common chronic diseases in the United States. One in six children aged 6–11 years and one in four adults have untreated cavities. Untreated cavities can cause pain and infections that may lead to problems eating, speaking, and learning. On average, 34 million school hours are lost each year because of unplanned (emergency) dental care, and almost $46 billion is lost in productivity due to dental disease.

RISK FACTORS

Cigarette Smoking

More than 16 million Americans have at least one disease caused by cigarette smoking. This amounts to more than $240 billion in health-care spending that could be reduced every year if we could prevent young people from starting to smoke and help every person who smokes to quit.

Physical Inactivity

Not getting enough physical activity comes with high health and financial costs. It can lead to heart disease, type 2 diabetes, some cancers, and obesity. Physical inactivity also costs the nation $117 billion a year for related health care.

Excessive Alcohol Use

Excessive alcohol use is responsible for 178,000 deaths in the United States each year, including one in five deaths among adults aged 20–49 years. Binge drinking is responsible for over one-third of these deaths. In 2010, excessive alcohol use cost the U.S. economy

$249 billion, or $2.05 a drink, and $2 of every $5 of these costs were paid by the public. Three-quarters of these costs were due to binge drinking.[1]

[1] "Health and Economic Costs of Chronic Conditions," Centers for Disease Control and Prevention (CDC), July 12, 2024. Available online. URL: www.cdc.gov/chronic-disease/data-research/facts-stats/index.html. Accessed September 30, 2024.

Chapter 20 | **Preventive Health Services and Screening**

Chapter Contents

Section 20.1 | Preventive Services and Special Health Needs in Marketplace Plans

COVERAGE OF MARKETPLACE HEALTH INSURANCE PLANS

Marketplace health insurance plans cover 10 essential health benefits, ensuring comprehensive care for enrolled individuals. These benefits include:

- **Ambulatory patient services.** Outpatient care received without being admitted to a hospital.
- **Emergency services.** Immediate care for urgent medical needs.
- **Hospitalization.** Services related to surgery and overnight stays.
- **Pregnancy, maternity, and newborn care.** Coverage before and after birth.
- **Mental health and substance use disorder services.** Includes behavioral health treatment, such as counseling and psychotherapy.
- **Prescription drugs.** Coverage for necessary medications.
- **Rehabilitative and habilitative services and devices.** These services and devices help individuals with injuries, disabilities, or chronic conditions regain or acquire mental and physical skills.
- **Laboratory services.** Testing and diagnostic services.
- **Preventive and wellness services and chronic disease management.** Services aimed at disease prevention and management.
- **Pediatric services.** Includes oral and vision care for children (adult dental and vision coverage are not essential health benefits).

ADDITIONAL BENEFITS

Plans must also include the following benefits:

- birth control coverage
- breastfeeding coverage

Essential health benefits represent minimum requirements for all Marketplace plans. Specific services covered in each broad benefit category can vary based on state requirements. Plans may offer additional benefits, including:

- dental coverage
- vision coverage
- medical management programs, for specific needs such as weight management, back pain, and diabetes

PREVENTIVE HEALTH SERVICES

Most health plans must cover a set of preventive services—such as vaccinations and screening tests—at no cost to you. This includes plans available through the Health Insurance Marketplace®. These services are free only when delivered by a doctor or other provider in your plan's network.

All Marketplace health plans and many other plans must cover the following list of preventive services without charging you a copayment or coinsurance, even if you haven't met your yearly deductible.

Preventive Care Benefits for Adults

Marketplace health plans must provide:

- abdominal aortic aneurysm one-time screening for men of specified ages who have ever smoked
- alcohol misuse screening and counseling
- aspirin use to prevent cardiovascular disease and colorectal cancer for adults aged 50–59 years with high cardiovascular risk
- blood pressure screening
- cholesterol screening for adults of certain ages or at higher risk
- colorectal cancer screening for adults aged 45–75
- depression screening
- diabetes (type 2) screening for adults aged 40–70 years who are overweight or obese
- diet counseling for adults at higher risk for chronic disease

- falls prevention (with exercise or physical therapy and vitamin D use) for adults aged 65 years and over living in a community setting
- hepatitis B screening for people at high risk, including individuals from countries with a 2 percent or more prevalence of hepatitis B, and U.S.-born individuals not vaccinated as infants with at least one parent born in a region with an 8 percent or more prevalence of hepatitis B
- hepatitis C screening for adults aged 18–79 years
- HIV screening for everyone aged 15–65, and for other ages at increased risk
- immunizations for adults
- lung cancer screening for adults aged 50–80 at high risk for lung cancer due to heavy smoking or having quit in the past 15 years
- obesity screening and counseling
- PrEP (pre-exposure prophylaxis) HIV prevention medication for HIV-negative adults at high risk for getting HIV through sex or injection drug use
- sexually transmitted infection (STI) prevention counseling for adults at higher risk
- statin preventive medication for adults aged 40–75 at high risk
- syphilis screening for adults at higher risk
- tobacco use screening for all adults and cessation interventions for tobacco users
- tuberculosis screening for certain adults without symptoms at high risk

Services for Pregnant Women or Women Who May Become Pregnant

Marketplace health plans must provide:

- breastfeeding support and counseling from trained providers and access to breastfeeding supplies for pregnant and nursing women
- birth control

- folic acid supplements for women who may become pregnant
- gestational diabetes screening for women 24 weeks pregnant or later and those at high risk of developing gestational diabetes
- gonorrhea screening for all women at higher risk
- hepatitis B screening for pregnant women at their first prenatal visit
- maternal depression screening for mothers at well-baby visits
- preeclampsia prevention and screening for pregnant women with high blood pressure
- Rh incompatibility screening for all pregnant women and follow-up testing for those at higher risk
- syphilis screening
- tobacco intervention and counseling for pregnant tobacco users
- urinary tract or other infection screening

Coverage for Children's Preventive Health Services

Marketplace plans cover preventive health services for children, including:

- alcohol, tobacco, and drug use assessments for adolescents
- autism screening for children at 18 and 24 months
- behavioral assessments for children
- bilirubin concentration screening for newborns
- blood pressure screening for children
- blood screening for newborns
- depression screening for adolescents beginning routinely at age 12
- developmental screening for children under age 3
- dyslipidemia screening for all children once between 9 and 11 years and once between 17 and 21 years, and for children at higher risk of lipid disorders
- fluoride supplements for children without fluoride in their water source

- fluoride varnish for all infants and children as soon as teeth are present
- gonorrhea preventive medication for the eyes of all newborns
- hearing screening for all newborns and regular screenings for children and adolescents as recommended by their provider
- height, weight, and body mass index (BMI) measurements taken regularly for all children
- hematocrit or hemoglobin screening for all children
- hemoglobinopathies or sickle cell screening for newborns
- hepatitis B screening for adolescents at higher risk
- HIV screening for adolescents at higher risk
- hypothyroidism screening for newborns
- immunizations for children from birth to age 18
- lead screening for children at risk of exposure
- obesity screening and counseling
- oral health risk assessment for young children from 6 months to 6 years
- phenylketonuria (PKU) screening for newborns
- PrEP (pre-exposure prophylaxis) HIV prevention medication for HIV-negative adolescents at high risk for getting HIV through sex or injection drug use
- sexually transmitted infection (STI) prevention counseling and screening for adolescents at higher risk
- tuberculin testing for children at higher risk of tuberculosis
- vision screening for all children
- well-baby and well-child visits[1]

[1] "Preventive Health Services," Centers for Medicare & Medicaid Services (CMS), April 18, 2024. Available online. URL: www.healthcare.gov/coverage/preventive-care-benefits. Accessed September 30, 2024.

Section 20.2 | National Breast and Cervical Cancer Early Detection Program

Through the National Breast and Cervical Cancer Early Detection Program (NBCCEDP), the Centers for Disease Control and Prevention (CDC) helps individuals with low incomes who do not have adequate insurance gain access to timely breast and cervical cancer screening, diagnostic, and treatment services.

PURPOSE

To improve access to breast and cervical cancer screening, Congress passed the Breast and Cervical Cancer Mortality Prevention Act of 1990, which directed the CDC to create the NBCCEDP. The program funds 71 award recipients across the United States.

In 1993, Congress amended the act with the Preventive Health Amendments of 1993 to authorize the CDC to fund American Indian and Alaska Native tribes and tribal organizations through the NBCCEDP. In 2000, Congress passed the Breast and Cervical Cancer Prevention and Treatment Act, allowing states to offer treatment access through Medicaid to those diagnosed with cancer in the NBCCEDP. In 2001, with the passage of the Native American Breast and Cervical Cancer Treatment Technical Amendment Act, Congress clarified that this option also applies to American Indian and Alaska Native women eligible for health services provided by the Indian Health Service or by a tribal organization.

Through the NBCCEDP, the CDC assists those with low incomes who do not have adequate insurance in gaining timely access to breast and cervical cancer screening, diagnostic, and treatment services. The program also provides patient navigation services to help overcome barriers and ensure timely access to quality care.

In addition to funding screening and diagnostic services for those eligible, the NBCCEDP focuses on factors at the interpersonal, organizational, community, and policy levels that influence screening. The program supports the use of population-based approaches to improve systems that increase high-quality breast and cervical cancer screening. These include:

- implementing evidence-based interventions in health systems
- connecting eligible individuals in the community to screening services
- informing policies that increase access to cancer screening[1]

Figure 20.1 illustrates the percentage of individuals receiving cervical cancer services in the United States, categorized by race and ethnicity.

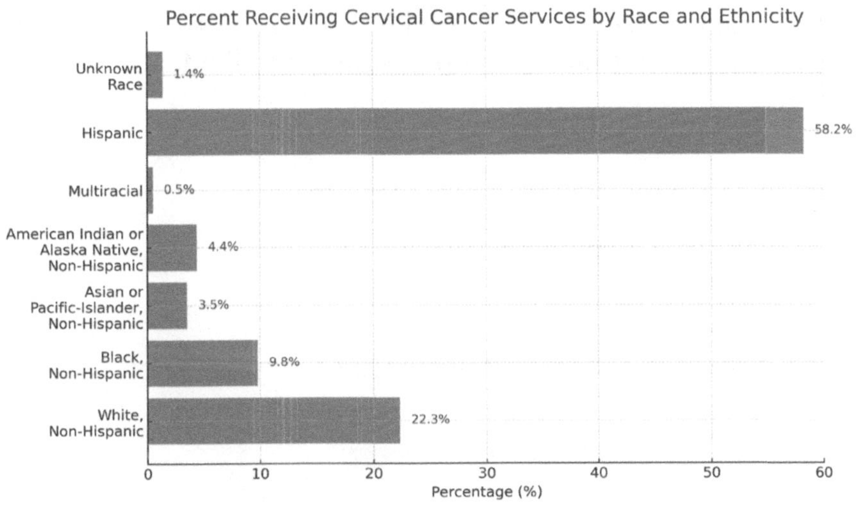

Figure 20.1. Percent Receiving Cervical Cancer Services by Race and Ethnicity

Centers for Disease Control and Prevention (CDC)

[1] "About the National Breast and Cervical Cancer Early Detection Program," Centers for Disease Control and Prevention (CDC), September 19, 2024. Available online. URL: www.cdc.gov/breast-cervical-cancer-screening/about/index.html. Accessed September 30, 2024.

Figure 20.2 shows the distribution of cervical cancer service utilization by age group, with the highest percentages among individuals aged 40–64. It highlights that people aged 50–64 have the highest service utilization, followed closely by those aged 40–49, with lower percentages among younger individuals and those in other age categories.

Figure 20.3 illustrates the percentage of individuals receiving breast cancer services in the United States, broken down by race and ethnicity. Hispanic individuals represent the largest group utilizing these services, followed by non-Hispanic white and non-Hispanic Black populations, with smaller percentages for other racial and ethnic groups.

Figure 20.4 shows the distribution of breast cancer service utilization by age group, with the majority of services received by individuals aged 50–64. It highlights that this age group accounts for the largest percentage, followed by those aged 40–49, with significantly lower percentages among younger individuals and those over 65.

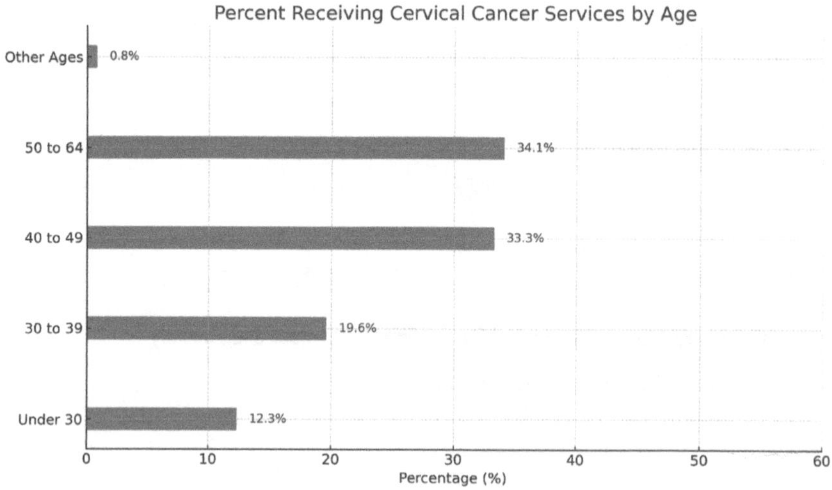

Figure 20.2. Percent Receiving Cervical Cancer Services by Age

Centers for Disease Control and Prevention (CDC)

Preventive Health Services and Screening

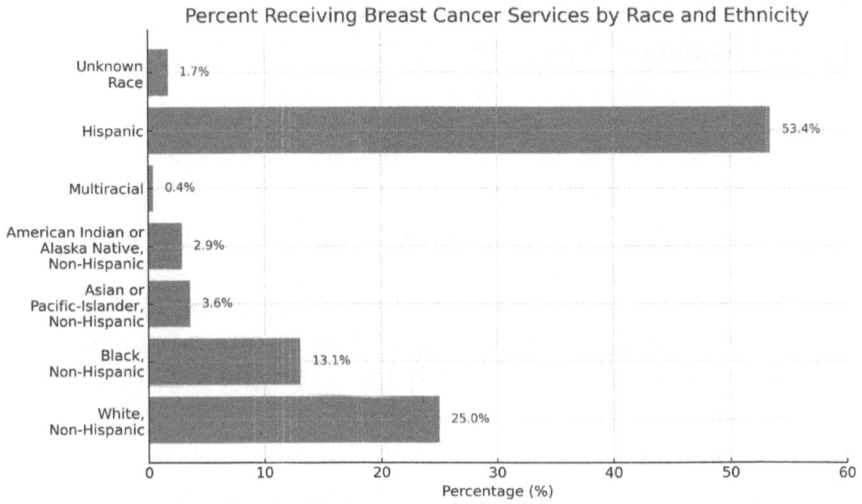

Figure 20.3. Percent Receiving Breast Cancer Services by Race and Ethnicity
Centers for Disease Control and Prevention (CDC)

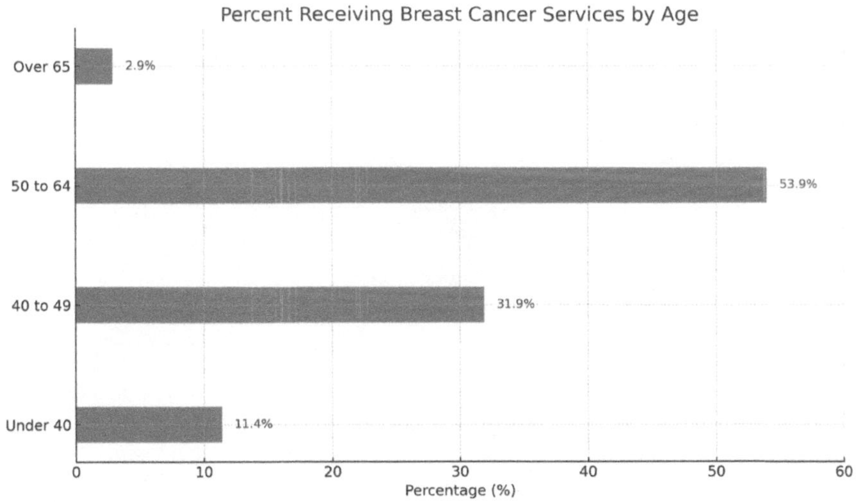

Figure 20.4. Percent Receiving Breast Cancer Services by Age
Centers for Disease Control and Prevention (CDC)

FIND A SCREENING PROGRAM NEAR YOU

Are You Eligible for Free or Low-Cost Screenings?

You may be eligible for free or low-cost screenings if you meet the following criteria:

- Have no insurance, or your insurance does not cover screening exams.
- Have a yearly income at or below 250 percent of the federal poverty level.
- Are aged 40–64 for breast cancer screening or 21–64 for cervical cancer screening (certain women who are younger or older may qualify for screening services).

Select a Program

Select a state, territory, or tribe to see the award recipient's contact information and screening program summaries (www.cdc.gov/breast-cervical-cancer-screening/about/screenings.html).[2]

[2] "Find a Screening Program Near You," Centers for Disease Control and Prevention (CDC), January 10, 2024. Available online. URL: www.cdc.gov/breast-cervical-cancer-screening/about/screenings.html. Accessed September 30, 2024.

Chapter 21 | Disparities in Emergency Department Usage

EMERGENCY DEPARTMENT VISIT STATISTICS

In 2021, 140 million emergency department (ED) visits occurred in the United States. During that year, approximately 4 percent of children had two or more ED visits in the past 12 months, and 18 percent of adults had visited the ED in the past 12 months. This analysis, based on data from the 2021 National Hospital Ambulatory Medical Care Survey (NHAMCS), provides characteristics of ED visits by age group, sex, race and ethnicity, insurance status, and mentions of coronavirus 2019 (COVID-19).

KEY FINDINGS FROM THE NATIONAL HOSPITAL AMBULATORY MEDICAL CARE SURVEY

- The overall emergency department (ED) visit rate was 43 visits per 100 people in 2021.
- The ED visit rates were highest for infants under 1 year (103 visits per 100 infants) and adults aged 75 and over (66 visits per 100 people).
- The ED visit rate for Black or African-American non-Hispanic people (81 visits per 100 people) was the highest among the selected racial and ethnic groups.
- The ED visit rate for patients with private insurance was the lowest compared with all other primary expected sources of payment, and the rate for patients with Medicaid was the highest.
- In 2021, a COVID-19 diagnosis was confirmed for 3.8 percent of all ED patient visits.

WHAT WAS THE EMERGENCY DEPARTMENT VISIT RATE IN 2021, AND DID VISIT RATES VARY BY AGE?

- The total ED visit rate was 43 visits per 100 people in 2021 (see Figure 21.1).
- The ED visit rate was highest for infants under 1 year (103 visits per 100 infants), followed by adults aged 75 and over (66 visits per 100 people). These rates were higher than for all other age groups.
- The ED visit rates were similar for patients in age groups between ages 1 year and 74 years, ranging from 36 to 45 visits per 100 people.

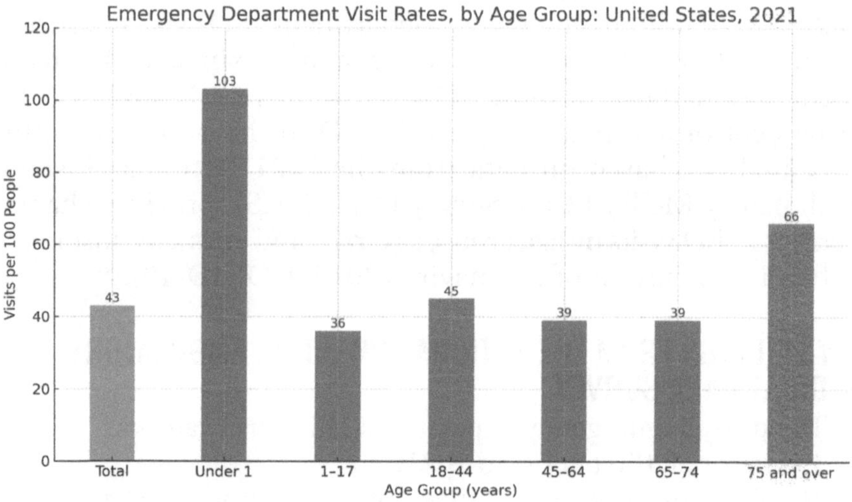

Figure 21.1. Emergency Department Visit Rates, by Age Group: United States, 2021

Centers for Disease Control and Prevention (CDC)
Source: National Center for Health Statistics, National Hospital Ambulatory Medical Care Survey, 2021.

DID EMERGENCY DEPARTMENT VISIT RATES VARY BY SEX OR RACE AND ETHNICITY?

- The 2021 ED visit rate for females (46 visits per 100 females) was similar to the ED visit rate for males (40 visits per 100 males; see Figure 21.2).

Disparities in Emergency Department Usage

- In 2021, the ED visit rate was highest for Black or African-American non-Hispanic (subsequently, Black) people (81 visits per 100 people) compared with white non-Hispanic (subsequently, white) people (41 visits per 100 people); Hispanic people (36 visits per 100 people); and people of other non-Hispanic races (subsequently, other races; 17 visits per 100 people). Rates were lowest among other races.

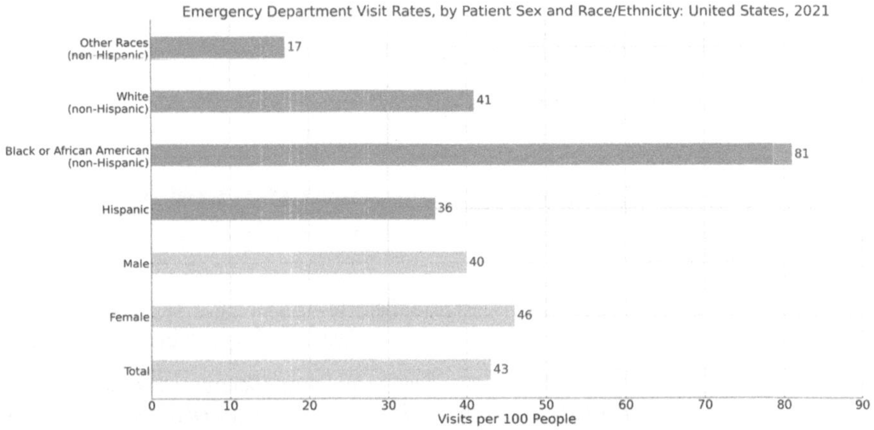

Figure 21.2. Emergency Department Visit Rates, by Patient Sex and Race and Ethnicity: United States, 2021

Centers for Disease Control and Prevention (CDC)
Source: National Center for Health Statistics, National Hospital Ambulatory Medical Care Survey, 2021.

WHAT WERE THE EMERGENCY DEPARTMENT VISIT RATES FOR EACH PRIMARY EXPECTED SOURCE OF PAYMENT, AND DID THESE RATES VARY?

- The ED visit rate was highest for patients with Medicaid, Children's Health Insurance Program (CHIP), or other state-based programs (89 visits per 100 people) and lowest for patients with private insurance (22 visits per 100 people; see Figure 21.3).
- The ED visit rates for patients with Medicare (46 visits per 100 people), patients with other primary expected sources

of payment (43 visits per 100 people), and patients with no insurance (33 visits per 100 people) were not significantly different.

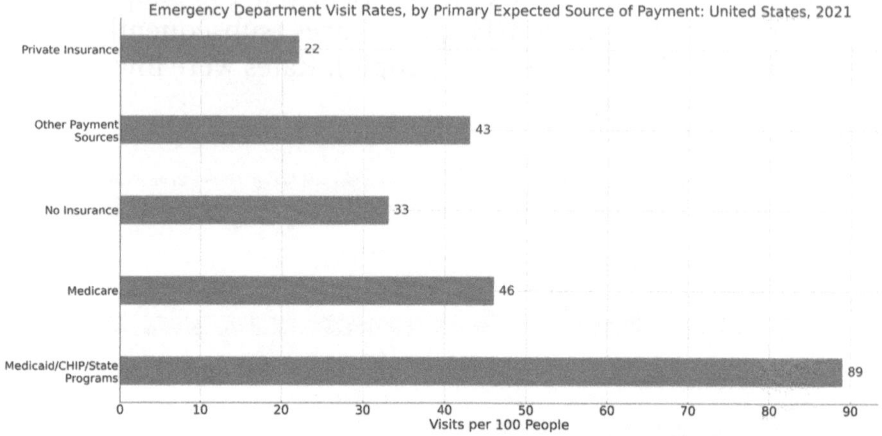

Figure 21.3. Emergency Department Visit Rates, by Primary Expected Source of Payment: United States, 2021

Centers for Disease Control and Prevention (CDC)
Source: National Center for Health Statistics, National Hospital Ambulatory Medical Care Survey, 2021.

WHAT PERCENTAGE OF EMERGENCY DEPARTMENT VISITS WERE RELATED TO COVID-19?

- An estimated 14.2 percent of all ED visits in 2021 had any mention of COVID-19 (see Figure 21.4).
- COVID-19 cases were confirmed at 3.8 percent of ED visits.
- 8.8 percent of ED visits included a COVID-19 test or screening, and 3.2 percent of visits included suspected exposure to COVID-19.[1]

[1] "Emergency Department Visit Rates by Selected Characteristics: United States, 2021," Centers for Disease Control and Prevention (CDC), August 2023. Available online. URL: www.cdc.gov/nchs/data/databriefs/db478.pdf. Accessed September 30, 2024.

Disparities in Emergency Department Usage

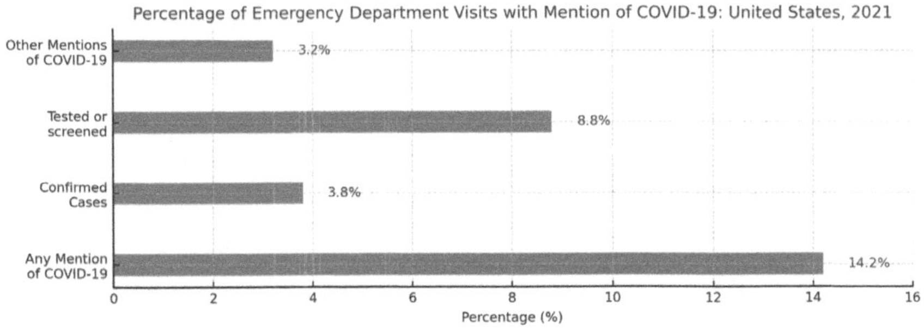

Figure 21.4. Percentage of Emergency Department Visits with Mention of COVID-19: United States, 2021

Centers for Disease Control and Prevention (CDC)
Source: National Center for Health Statistics, National Hospital Ambulatory Medical Care Survey, 2021.

Part 4 | Genetics/ Genomics and Demographics

Chapter 22 | **Understanding Genetics and Genomics**

Chapter Contents

Section 22.1 | The Science of Genes, Chromosomes, and Health

WHAT IS A GENE?

A gene is the basic physical and functional unit of heredity. Genes are made up of DNA (deoxyribonucleic acid). Some genes act as instructions to make molecules called "proteins." However, many genes do not code for proteins. In humans, genes vary in size from a few hundred DNA bases to more than 2 million bases. An international research effort called the "Human Genome Project," which worked to determine the sequence of the human genome and identify the genes that it contains, estimated that humans have between 20,000 and 25,000 genes.

Every person has two copies of each gene, one inherited from each parent. Most genes are the same in all people, but a few genes (less than 1 percent of the total) are slightly different between people. Alleles are forms of the same gene with small differences in their sequence of DNA bases. These small differences contribute to each person's unique physical features.

Scientists keep track of genes by giving them unique names. Because gene names can be long, genes are also assigned symbols, which are short combinations of letters (and sometimes numbers) that represent an abbreviated version of the gene name. For example, a gene on chromosome 7 that has been associated with cystic fibrosis (CF) is called the "cystic fibrosis transmembrane conductance regulator"; its symbol is *CFTR*.

WHAT IS A CHROMOSOME?

In the nucleus of each cell, the DNA molecule is packaged into thread-like structures called "chromosomes." Each chromosome is made up of DNA tightly coiled many times around proteins called "histones" that support its structure.

Chromosomes are not visible in the cell's nucleus—not even under a microscope—when the cell is not dividing. However, the DNA that makes up chromosomes becomes more tightly packed during cell division and is then visible under a microscope. Most of what researchers know about chromosomes was learned by observing chromosomes during cell division.

Each chromosome has a constriction point called the "centromere," which divides it into two sections, or "arms." The short arm of the chromosome is labeled the "p arm." The long arm of the chromosome is labeled the "q arm." The location of the centromere on each chromosome gives the chromosome its characteristic shape and can help describe the location of specific genes.

WHAT IS A GENE VARIANT AND HOW DO VARIANTS OCCUR?

A gene variant is a permanent change in the DNA sequence that makes up a gene. This type of genetic change used to be known as a "gene mutation," but because changes in DNA do not always cause disease, it is thought that "gene variant" is a more accurate term. Variants can affect one or more DNA building blocks (nucleotides) in a gene.

Gene variants can be inherited from a parent or occur during a person's lifetime:

- **Inherited (or hereditary) variants are passed from parent to child and are present throughout a person's life in virtually every cell in the body.** These variants are also called "germline variants" because they are present in the parent's egg or sperm cells, which are also called "germ cells." When an egg and a sperm cell unite, the resulting fertilized egg cell contains DNA from both parents. Any variants that are present in that DNA will be present in the cells of the child that grows from the fertilized egg.
- **Noninherited variants occur at some time during a person's life and are present only in certain cells, not in every cell in the body.** Because noninherited variants typically occur in somatic cells (cells other than sperm and egg cells), they are often referred to as "somatic variants." These variants cannot be passed to the next generation. Noninherited variants can be caused by environmental factors such as ultraviolet

radiation from the sun or can occur if an error is made as DNA copies itself during cell division.

HOW CAN GENE VARIANTS AFFECT HEALTH AND DEVELOPMENT?

To function correctly, each cell depends on thousands of proteins to do their jobs in the right places at the right times. Sometimes, gene variants (also known as "mutations") prevent one or more proteins from working properly. By changing a gene's instructions for making a protein, a variant can cause a protein to malfunction or not be produced at all. When a variant alters a protein that plays a critical role in the body, it can disrupt normal development or cause a health condition. A condition caused by variants in one or more genes is called a "genetic disorder."

In some cases, gene variants are so severe that they prevent an embryo from surviving until birth. These changes occur in genes that are essential for development and often disrupt an embryo's development in its earliest stages. Because these variants have very serious effects, they are incompatible with life.

It is important to note that genes themselves do not cause disease—genetic disorders are caused by variants that alter or eliminate a gene's function. For example, when people say that someone has "the cystic fibrosis gene," they are usually referring to a version of the *CFTR* gene that contains a variant that causes the disease. All people, including those without cystic fibrosis, have a version of the *CFTR* gene.

DO ALL GENE VARIANTS AFFECT HEALTH AND DEVELOPMENT?

No; only a small percentage of variants cause genetic disorders—most have no impact on health or development. For example, some variants alter a gene's DNA sequence but do not change the function of the protein made from the gene.

Often, gene variants that could cause a genetic disorder are repaired by certain enzymes before the gene is expressed and an altered protein is produced. Each cell has a number of pathways through which enzymes recognize and repair errors in DNA.

Because DNA can be changed or damaged in many ways, DNA repair is an important process by which the body protects itself from disease.

A very small percentage of all variants actually have a positive effect. These variants lead to new versions of proteins that help an individual better adapt to changes in his or her environment. For example, a beneficial variant could result in a protein that protects an individual and future generations from a new strain of bacteria.

Because a person's genetic code can have many variants with no effect on health, diagnosing genetic disorders can be difficult. When determining if a gene variant is associated with a genetic disorder, the variant is evaluated using scientific research to date, such as information on how the variant affects the function or production of the protein made from the gene and previous variant classification data. The variant is then classified on a spectrum based on how likely it is to lead to the disorder.

CAN A CHANGE IN THE NUMBER OF GENES AFFECT HEALTH AND DEVELOPMENT?

People have two copies of most genes, one copy inherited from each parent. In some cases, however, the number of copies varies—meaning that a person can have one, three, or more copies of particular genes. Less commonly, both copies of a gene may be missing. These types of genetic differences are known as "copy number variations" (CNV).

Copy number variation results from insertions, deletions, and duplications of large segments of DNA that are at least one thousand nucleotides (also called "1 kilobase" or "1 kb") in length. These segments are often big enough to include whole genes. Variations in gene copy number can influence the activity of genes and the functioning of proteins made from them, which may affect body processes.

Copy number variation accounts for a significant amount of genetic difference between people. More than 10 percent of the human genome appears to contain differences in gene copy number. While much of this variation does not affect health or development, some differences influence a person's risk of disease—particularly some types of cancer—or response to certain drugs.

CAN CHANGES IN THE STRUCTURE OF CHROMOSOMES AFFECT HEALTH AND DEVELOPMENT?

Changes in the structure of chromosomes can cause problems with the growth, development, and function of the body's systems. These changes can affect many genes along the chromosome and disrupt the proteins made from those genes.

Structural changes can occur during the formation of egg or sperm cells, in early fetal development, or in any cell after birth. Pieces of DNA can be rearranged within one chromosome or transferred between two or more chromosomes. The effects of structural changes depend on their size and location, whether gene function is interrupted, and whether any genetic material is gained or lost. Some changes cause health problems, while others may have no effect on a person's health.[1]

Section 22.2 | **The Human Genome Project**

The Human Genome Project was a large, well-organized, and highly collaborative international effort that generated the first sequence of the human genome and that of several additional well-studied organisms. Carried out from 1990 to 2003, it was one of the most ambitious and important scientific endeavors in human history. In 2003, the Human Genome Project produced a genome sequence that accounted for over 90 percent of the human genome. It was as close to complete as the technologies for sequencing DNA (deoxyribonucleic acid) allowed at the time.

The project was critical for advancing policies and earning increased support for the open sharing of scientific data. Concerns and questions about sequencing the human genome helped usher

[1] MedlinePlus, "Help Me Understand Genetics," National Institutes of Health (NIH), July 14, 2015. Available online. URL: www.medlineplus.gov/download/genetics/understanding/primer.pdf. Accessed September 25, 2024.

in a greater emphasis on ethics in biomedical research. The project was atypical for biomedical research in that the researchers' work was driven by a desire to explore an unknown part of the biological world, as opposed to first formulating a theory or hypothesis.

WHAT WERE THE GOALS OF THE HUMAN GENOME PROJECT?

A special committee of the U.S. National Academy of Sciences outlined the original goals for the Human Genome Project in 1988, which included sequencing the entire human genome in addition to the genomes of several carefully selected nonhuman organisms.

Eventually, the list of organisms came to include the bacterium *E. coli*, baker's yeast, fruit fly, nematode, and mouse. The project's architects and participants hoped the resulting information would usher in a new era for biomedical research, and its goals and related strategic plans were updated periodically throughout the project.

In part due to a deliberate focus on technology development, the Human Genome Project ultimately exceeded its initial set of goals, doing so by 2003, two years ahead of its originally projected completion in 2005. Many of the project's achievements were beyond what scientists thought possible in 1988.

WHAT IS DNA SEQUENCING?

DNA sequencing involves determining the exact order of the bases in DNA—the As, Cs, Gs, and Ts that make up segments of DNA. Because the Human Genome Project aimed to sequence all the DNA (i.e., the genome) of a set of organisms, significant effort was made to improve the methods for DNA sequencing.

Ultimately, the project used one particular method for DNA sequencing, called "Sanger DNA sequencing," but first greatly advanced this basic method through a series of major technical innovations.

WHOSE GENOME WAS SEQUENCED BY THE HUMAN GENOME PROJECT?

The human genome sequence generated by the Human Genome Project was actually a patchwork of multiple people whose identities were intentionally made anonymous to protect their privacy.

However, the majority of the sequence came from one person of blended ancestry. Specifically, 70 percent of the original reference human genome sequence was generated from that individual's DNA, with the remaining 30 percent coming from a combination of 19 other people of mostly European ancestry.

HOW WAS THE DNA COLLECTED BY THE HUMAN GENOME PROJECT?

Most of the original human genome sequence came from volunteers living in Buffalo, New York. Researchers at the Roswell Park Cancer Institute, located in Buffalo, were experts at preparing the DNA in a form that could be used for sequencing the human genome.

The researchers recruited volunteer donors through public advertisements. They then acquired informed consent from these volunteers and collected blood samples, from which they extracted DNA.

DID THE HUMAN GENOME PROJECT PRODUCE A PERFECTLY COMPLETE GENOME SEQUENCE?

No. Throughout the Human Genome Project, researchers continually improved their DNA sequencing methods. However, they were limited in their abilities to determine the sequence of some stretches of human DNA (e.g., particularly complex or highly repetitive DNA).

In June 2000, the International Human Genome Sequencing Consortium announced that it had produced a draft human genome sequence that accounted for 90 percent of the human genome. The draft sequence contained more than 150,000 areas where the DNA sequence was unknown because it could not be determined accurately (known as "gaps").

In April 2003, the consortium announced that it had generated an essentially complete human genome sequence, which was significantly improved from the draft sequence. Specifically, it accounted for 92 percent of the human genome and less than 400 gaps; it was also more accurate.

On March 31, 2022, the Telomere-to-Telomere (T2T) consortium announced that it had filled in the remaining gaps and produced the first truly complete human genome sequence (www.genome.gov/about-genomics/telomere-to-telomere).

HOW DID THE HUMAN GENOME PROJECT AFFECT BIOLOGICAL RESEARCH IN GENERAL?

The Human Genome Project demonstrated that production-oriented, discovery-driven scientific inquiry—which did not involve investigating a specific hypothesis or directly answering preformed questions—could be remarkably valuable and beneficial to the broader scientific community.

The project was also a successful example of "big science" in biomedical research. The magnitude of the technological challenges prompted the Human Genome Project to assemble interdisciplinary groups from across the world, involving experts in engineering, biology, and computer science, among other areas. It also required the work to be concentrated in a modest number of major centers to maximize economies of scale.

Before the Human Genome Project, the biomedical research community viewed projects of such scale with deep skepticism. These kinds of massive scientific undertakings have become more commonplace and well-accepted based in part on the success of the Human Genome Project.[1]

Section 22.3 | Genetic Factors in Disease and Health

WHAT ARE GENETIC DISORDERS?

Genetic disorders are health problems that happen because of some type of abnormality in a person's genetic material. There are several

[1] "Human Genome Project," National Human Genome Research Institute (NHGRI), June 13, 2024. Available online. URL: www.genome.gov/about-genomics/educational-resources/fact-sheets/human-genome-project. Accessed September 25, 2024.

types of genetic disorders. In some cases, a genetic change in a single gene can cause someone to have a disease or condition. In other cases, the gene does not have a genetic change, but a person has more or fewer copies of the gene than most people, and this causes a disease or condition. Some diseases or conditions occur when a person does not have the same number of chromosomes as most people or has part of a chromosome that is missing, extra, or not in the right place.

Most genetic disorders result from the combination of many genetic changes acting together with a person's behaviors and environment. These are sometimes called "complex conditions."

SINGLE GENE DISORDERS

Deoxyribonucleic acid (DNA) contains the instructions for making your body work. DNA is made up of two strands that wind around each other. Each DNA strand includes chemicals called "nitrogen bases—T (thymine)," "A (adenine)," "C (cytosine)," and "G (guanine)"—that make up the DNA code. Genes are specific sections of DNA that have instructions for making proteins. Proteins make up most of the parts of your body and make your body work the right way.

Some diseases and conditions happen when a person has a genetic change (sometimes called a "mutation") in one of their genes. These types of diseases are called "single gene disorders." Sometimes, what happens is that one of the DNA bases is changed. For example, part of a gene that usually has the sequence TAC is changed to the sequence TTC. This can change the way the gene works, for example, by changing the protein that is made. In other cases, one or more of the bases in the DNA sequence are missing altogether, or there are extra bases.

Genetic changes can be passed down to a child from their parents. When this happens, the disease or condition is called "hereditary" or "inherited." The changes can happen for the first time in the process of making the sperm or egg or early in development, so the child will have the genetic change, but the parents will not.

Single gene disorders that affect a gene on one of the 22 autosomal chromosome pairs are called "autosomal disorders." Disorders that affect the sex chromosome are called "X-linked disorders." Disorders are further described according to whether the affected genetic change is dominant or recessive.

For some diseases and conditions, everyone who inherits the genetic change will have the disease or condition, but how serious it is can vary from person to person. In other cases, people who have the genetic change will be more likely to develop the disease or condition, but some of them will never develop it.

Autosomal Dominant

With autosomal dominant diseases or conditions, a person only needs a genetic change in one copy of the gene to have the disease. If one parent has an autosomal dominant disease or condition, each child has a 50 percent (1 in 2) chance of inheriting the genetic change that causes the condition.

Examples of autosomal dominant conditions include hereditary breast and ovarian cancer caused by genetic changes (mutations) to the *BRCA1* and *BRCA2* genes; Lynch syndrome; and familial hypercholesterolemia.

Autosomal Recessive

With autosomal recessive diseases or conditions, a person needs a genetic change in both copies of the gene to have the disease or condition. While a person with a genetic change in only one copy of the gene will not have the disease or condition, they can still pass the genetic change down to their children. These parents are sometimes called "carriers" of the disease because they "carry" the genetic change that causes the disease or condition but do not have the disease themselves.

A parent who is a carrier of a disease has a 50 percent (1 in 2) chance of passing the gene with the genetic change on to each of their children. If both parents are carriers of the disease, each child has a 25 percent (1 in 4) chance of inheriting two genes with the genetic change and thus of having the disease. Carrier screening looks for autosomal recessive genetic changes in parents to see if they could have a child with the disease or condition.

Examples of autosomal recessive disorders are sickle cell disease (SCD) and cystic fibrosis (CF).

X-Linked

Females have two X chromosomes, and males have one X chromosome and one Y chromosome. Each daughter gets an X from her mother and an X from her father, and each son gets an X from his mother and a Y from his father.

Some diseases or conditions happen when a gene on the X chromosome has a genetic change. Because males only have one copy of all the genes on the X chromosome, they are much more likely to be affected by X-linked genetic disorders than females. A female with a genetic change on only one of her two X chromosomes may not have the disease or condition at all. However, in some cases, females with a genetic change on one of their X chromosomes can have the disease or condition, but it is often a milder form of the disease than usually occurs in males.

Because males inherit an X chromosome from their mother, a female with a genetic change on one copy of the gene has a 50 percent (1 in 2) chance of passing the genetic change on to each of her sons. Her sons could have the disease or condition even though she does not.

Examples of X-linked conditions include fragile X syndrome, Duchenne muscular dystrophy, and hereditary hemophilia.

CHROMOSOMAL ABNORMALITIES

Different Number of Chromosomes

People usually have 23 pairs of chromosomes, but sometimes, a person is born with a different number. Having an extra chromosome is called "trisomy," and missing a chromosome is called "monosomy."

For example, people with Down syndrome have an extra copy of chromosome 21. This extra copy changes the body's and brain's normal development and causes intellectual and physical problems for the person. Some disorders are caused by having a different number of sex chromosomes. For example, people with Turner syndrome usually have only one sex chromosome, an X. Women with Turner syndrome can have problems with growth and heart defects.

Changes in Chromosomes

Sometimes chromosomes are incomplete or shaped differently than usual. A small part of a chromosome is missing, and this is called a "deletion." A "translocation" occurs when part of one chromosome moves to another chromosome, and an "inversion" occurs when part of a chromosome is flipped over.

For example, people with Williams syndrome are missing a small part of chromosome 7. This deletion can result in intellectual disability and a distinctive facial appearance and personality.

COMPLEX CONDITIONS

Complex disorders are caused by genetic changes in many different genes working together with environmental factors. Environmental factors include exposures and behaviors such as air pollution, smoking, alcohol use, the amount of exercise a person gets, or the foods they eat. Having a family health history of a complex condition can make you more likely to have that condition yourself. However, genetic testing would not be recommended because there is not a single genetic change causing the condition that could be found by genetic testing.

Most chronic diseases, such as most cases of heart disease, cancer, diabetes, osteoporosis, and asthma, are complex disorders. So are most cases of developmental disabilities, such as autism spectrum disorder and attention-deficit/hyperactivity disorder (ADHD), and mental health conditions, such as depression and schizophrenia.

The vast amount of genetic information available has allowed researchers to develop methods to study which types of genetic changes are found more often in people with a given disease or condition. This allows researchers to estimate a person's risk for a particular disorder based on which genetic changes they have. This estimate is known as the "polygenic risk score."

Some important issues need to be considered before polygenic risk scores can be routinely used in health care and public health. Studies are looking at how useful polygenic risk scores are in real-life clinical practice. Information on how each gene change affects disease risk comes from population-level genetic studies. Addressing diversity in the development of polygenic risk scores is important because polygenic risk scores developed from studies in one population (such as people of Northern European ancestry) might not work as well for other populations (such as people of West African ancestry). Also, how each gene change affects the polygenic risk score varies from study to study.

Once polygenic risk scores are ready to be used routinely in clinical practice, public health efforts will be needed to address issues such as access, insurance coverage, and sharing of results across health systems.[1]

Section 22.4 | Exploring Gene-Environment Interactions in Public Health

GENE-ENVIRONMENT INTERACTION

"Gene-environment interaction" refers to the interplay of genes (and, more broadly, genome function) and the physical and social environment. These interactions influence the expression of phenotypes. For example, most human traits and diseases are influenced by how one or more genes interact in complex ways with environmental factors, such as:

- chemicals in the air or water
- nutrition
- ultraviolet radiation from the sun
- social context

[1] "Genetic Disorders," Centers for Disease Control and Prevention (CDC), May 15, 2024. Available online. URL: www.cdc.gov/genomics-and-health/about/genetic-disorders.html. Accessed September 28, 2024.

UNDERSTANDING GENE-ENVIRONMENT INTERACTIONS CAN IMPROVE PUBLIC HEALTH

Gene-environment interactions are situations in which the effect of environmental exposure on disease risk is different for people with different genotypes or, conversely, where the influence of a genotype on disease risk is different in people with different environmental exposures. Studies of gene-environment interactions can provide insights into the biological mechanisms of disease and could have public health implications.

One example of a gene-environment interaction involves the *NAT2* gene, smoking as the environmental factor, and bladder cancer. Tobacco smoking is a known risk factor for bladder cancer. According to the American Cancer Society, smokers are at least three times as likely to get bladder cancer as nonsmokers. Smokers with one variant in *NAT2* have a much higher risk of bladder cancer compared to smokers with a different variant. In other words, it is the combination, or interaction, of the genetic factor—*NAT2* variation—and the environmental factor—smoking behavior—that determines bladder cancer risk.[1]

Considering both genetic factors and environmental influences is vital for understanding health outcomes and disease prevention. Focusing on these elements separately paints an incomplete picture, according to Christine Ladd-Acosta, PhD, an epidemiologist at the Johns Hopkins Bloomberg School of Public Health.

During the Keystone Science Lecture, Ladd-Acosta outlined why and how to consider environmental exposure data alongside genetic information to help researchers achieve the following goals:

- Identify modifiable risk factors to promote prevention.
- Uncover biological mechanisms to develop new treatments.
- Find predictive biomarkers to improve diagnosis, prognosis, and treatment response.
- Provide population-level perspective to inform public health interventions.

[1] "Gene Environment Interaction," National Human Genome Research Institute (NHGRI), September 25, 2024. Available online. URL: www.genome.gov/genetics-glossary/Gene-Environment-Interaction. Accessed September 28, 2024.

Ladd-Acosta currently leads several federally funded research projects to investigate how genes and the environment contribute to health and disease, particularly neurodevelopmental conditions.

"Dr. Ladd-Acosta's research program tackles fundamental questions about the joint effects of genes and environment on autism and other health outcomes by harnessing the power of many large national and international epidemiology studies," said Cindy Lawler, PhD, who hosted the lecture and leads the Genes, Environment, and Health Branch at National Institute of Environmental Health Sciences (NIEHS).

REAL-WORLD EXAMPLES

Ladd-Acosta used several case studies to illustrate the value of combining genetic and environmental data. She began with the case of phenylketonuria, a disease that prevents the breakdown of the amino acid phenylalanine. The buildup of phenylalanine in the blood and brain damages the nervous system. Though caused by a rare genetic mutation, the condition is also, in part, environmental because symptoms only appear if mutation carriers eat food containing phenylalanine.

"Using this information, we can modify individual diet to prevent the symptoms from appearing," said Ladd-Acosta. "Public health initiatives that include universal genetic screening shortly after birth could help identify infants with specific variants that require treatment. Considering both genetic and environmental factors is crucial at a population-wide level."

Ladd-Acosta also noted that gene-environment interactions are crucial for understanding biological processes involved in health outcomes. For example, she called attention to the fact that certain mutations on the *CCR5* gene—which can confer resistance to HIV (human immunodeficiency virus)—have helped to shed light on the biological mechanism underlying this condition and possible avenues for therapeutic prevention and treatment.

"Scientists studying this gene variant found that carriers display a change in the structure of their cell membranes, which can prevent HIV from binding," said Ladd-Acosta. "This mechanism is now targeted for therapeutics, providing a really clear case of how studying the relationship between genes and environment can have a positive impact on health."

SUGGESTIONS FOR GENE-ENVIRONMENT STUDIES

In addition to emphasizing the value of this line of research, Ladd-Acosta also provided a set of suggestions for environmental health researchers to consider as part of their studies. These recommendations include practical tips, as well as knowledge gaps that need to be addressed.

- **Study design**. Develop larger datasets that include genetic, environmental, and outcome information derived from multiple studies.
- **Statistical methods**. Consider which statistical model is most appropriate for a particular hypothesis and whether tools such as machine learning could help.
- **Genomic analyses**. Conduct more genome-wide association studies to connect exposures, outcomes, and biological pathways, including studies of how genes influence exposure-response and how maternal genetics influence exposure during pregnancy.
- **Exposure measures**. Carry out more gene-environment chemical exposure studies, with particular attention to mixtures of toxic chemicals.

Ladd-Acosta stressed that more time, attention, and resources should be devoted to gene-environment research. She would also like to see increased efforts to diversify the types of participants included in studies and the range of topics being addressed.

"From 2008 to 2022, there was a major increase in gene-environment studies, but most focused on European individuals and very few other racial or ethnic categories," Ladd-Acosta said. "There is also very little research on the physical and built environment, including exposures that NIEHS is really interested in, such as toxic chemicals and pollutants."

To address this gap, Ladd-Acosta is co-leading an NIEHS-supported project to shed new light on gene-environment interaction in autism spectrum disorder (ASD) across a network of 18 sites and multiple studies. The "Combining Advances in Genomics and Environmental Science to Accelerate Actionable Research (GEARs) in ASD Network" is creating the infrastructure and processes to harmonize large-scale data on both genetics and the environment using novel statistical methods to improve understanding of the causes and consequences of ASD.[2]

[2] "Understanding Gene-Environment Interactions Can Improve Public Health," National Institute of Environmental Health Sciences (NIEHS), June 2024. Available online. URL: https://factor.niehs.nih.gov/2024/6/science-highlights/gene-environment. Accessed September 28, 2024.

Chapter 23 | Understanding Family Health History for Better Health Outcomes

THE IMPORTANCE OF KNOWING AND SHARING YOUR FAMILY HEALTH HISTORY

Knowing and acting on your family health history can be an important part of staying healthy. Family health history can help your health-care provider decide which screening tests and other interventions you need and when. For example, if you have a parent or sibling diagnosed with breast cancer before age 50, your health-care provider might refer you for cancer genetic counseling.

Whether you know a lot about your family's health history or only a little, take time to talk to your family about their health histories. It might not be easy. Your family members might not be used to discussing their diseases or might not want to talk. But starting the conversation is important. Remember, you are asking not just for your own health, but for the health of everyone in your family.

If you have a medical condition, such as cancer, heart disease, or diabetes, be sure to let your family members know about your diagnosis. If you have had genetic testing done, share your results with your family members. If you are one of the older members of your family, you may know more about diseases and health conditions in your family, especially in relatives who are no longer living. Be sure to share this information with your younger relatives so that you may all benefit from knowing this family health history information.

COLLECT AND SHARE YOUR FAMILY HEALTH HISTORY

Are you ready to collect your family health history but do not know where to start? Here is how:

- **Talk to your family.** Write down the names of your close blood relatives from both sides of the family: parents, siblings, half-siblings, grandparents, aunts, uncles, nieces, and nephews. Talk to these family members about what conditions they have or had and at what age the conditions were first diagnosed. You might think you know about all the conditions in your parents or siblings, but you might find out more information if you ask.
- **Ask questions.** To find out about your risk for chronic diseases, ask your relatives about which of these diseases they have had and when they were diagnosed. Questions can include:
  - Do you have any chronic diseases, such as heart disease or diabetes, or health conditions such as high blood pressure or high cholesterol?
  - Have you had any other serious diseases, such as cancer or stroke? What type of cancer?
  - How old were you when each of these diseases and health conditions were diagnosed? (If your relative does not remember the exact age, knowing the approximate age is still useful.)
  - What is our family's ancestry? From what countries did our ancestors come to the United States?
  - What were the causes and ages of death for relatives who have died?
- **Record the information and update it whenever you learn new family health history information.** My Family Health Portrait (https://cbiit.github.io/FHH/html/index.html) is a free web-based tool that helps you organize your family health history information and share it easily with your health-care provider and other family members.
- **Share family health history information with your health-care provider.** If you are concerned about

diseases that are common in your family, talk with your health-care provider at your next visit. Even if you do not know all of your family health history information, share what you do know. Family health history information, even if incomplete, can help your health-care provider decide which screening tests you need and when those tests should start.

- **Share your medical and family health history with your family members**. If you have a medical condition, such as cancer, heart disease, or diabetes, be sure to let your family members know about your diagnosis. If you have had genetic testing done, share your results with your family members. If you are one of the older members of your family, you may know more about diseases and health conditions in your family, especially in relatives who are no longer living. Be sure to share this information with your younger relatives so that you may all benefit from knowing this family health history information.

ACT ON YOUR FAMILY HEALTH HISTORY

Having a family health history of a disease does not mean that you or your family members will definitely get it. Knowing about your family health history of a disease can motivate you to take steps to lower your chances of getting the disease. You cannot change your family health history, but you can change unhealthy behaviors, such as smoking, not exercising or being active, and poor eating habits.

Talk with your health-care provider about steps you can take, including whether you should consider early screening for the disease. If you have a family history of disease, you may have the most to gain from lifestyle changes and screening tests.

What you can do if you have a family health history of the following conditions:

- **Colorectal cancer**. If you have a mother, father, sister, brother, or other close family member who had colorectal cancer before age 50 or have multiple close family members with colorectal cancer, talk to your health-care provider about whether you should start screening at a younger age, undergo screening more frequently, and use colonoscopy only instead of other tests. In some cases, your health-care provider may recommend that you have genetic counseling, and a genetic counselor may recommend genetic testing based on your family health history.

- **Breast or ovarian cancer.** If you have a parent, sibling, or child with breast cancer, follow current recommendations and start getting mammograms at age 40. If your relative was diagnosed with breast cancer before age 50, if you have a close relative with ovarian cancer, or if you have a male relative with breast cancer, your health-care provider might refer you for cancer genetic counseling to find out if genetic testing is right for you. In some cases, your health-care provider might recommend taking tamoxifen, raloxifene, or aromatase inhibitors, drugs that can decrease the risk of developing breast cancer in some women.
- **Heart disease.** If you have a family health history of heart disease, you can take steps to lower your chances of getting heart disease. These steps can include eating a healthy diet, being physically active, maintaining a healthy weight, not smoking, limiting your alcohol use, having any screening tests that your health-care provider recommends, and, in some cases, taking medication. If you or a family member has low-density lipoprotein (LDL) cholesterol levels over 190 mg/dL (or over 160 mg/dL in children), talk to your health-care provider about getting checked for familial hypercholesterolemia (FH), especially if you have a family health history of early heart disease or heart attacks.
- **Diabetes.** If your mother, father, brother, or sister has type 2 diabetes, you and your other family members could have prediabetes and are more likely to develop type 2 diabetes. While most people with type 2 diabetes are older adults, more and more children, teens, and

young adults are developing type 2 diabetes. However, there are important steps you and your children can take to prevent type 2 diabetes and reverse prediabetes if you have it. Take this test to find out if you or your family members could have prediabetes. Ask your health-care provider whether you need earlier screening for diabetes.

- **Osteoporosis.** This is a medical condition where bones become weak and are more likely to break. A family health history of osteoporosis is one of several factors that make you more likely to develop osteoporosis. For example, if you are a white woman whose mother or father fractured a hip, talk to your health-care provider about screening for osteoporosis earlier (at about age 55, compared with age 65 for most women).
- **Hereditary hemochromatosis.** It is a disorder in which the body can build up too much iron and can lead to serious liver damage and other problems. If you have a family member, especially a brother or sister, with hemochromatosis, you may be more likely to develop the condition yourself. Talk to your health-care provider about testing for hemochromatosis and whether you should take steps to lower the amount of iron in your body.[1]

[1] "Family Health History for Adults," Centers for Disease Control and Prevention (CDC), September 25, 2024. Available online. URL: www.cdc.gov/family-health-history/family-health-history-and-you/family-health-history-and-adults.html. Accessed September 28, 2024.

Chapter 24 | Predictive Analytics and Precision Public Health

WHAT IS PREDICTIVE ANALYTICS?

Predictive analytics in health is a set of analytic procedures that take existing information and forecast future probabilities of disease patterns, health behaviors, and other variables, using diverse data sources. Unlike traditional hypothesis-driven biomedical research, predictive analytics aims to tailor public health interventions to specific populations and individuals, a concept known as "precision public health." It uses statistical algorithms and comprehensive data (e.g., geospatial, burden of disease, demography, variation in community and health-care capacity, and more) to understand complex interrelationships between determinants of health and the variability of health care and public health service delivery.

HOW CAN PREDICTIVE ANALYTICS BE USED TO IMPROVE IMPLEMENTATION RESEARCH?

So far, predictive analytics has been used mostly as a business tool. This approach is not hypothesis-driven. Rather, the data drive the analytical direction seeking novel relationships. For population health, it is essential to understand how the community environment can support the implementation of health interventions. Predictive analytics can simulate a wide variety of clinical-, systems-, and population-level delivery interventions and also predict outcome measures and forecast results from selected intervention delivery scenarios.[1]

BIG DATA SCIENCE

The term “big data” refers to large data sets that require new methods for manipulation, analysis, and interpretation. Such data include genomic and other biomarkers, sociodemographic, environmental, geographic, and other information.

The abundance of these data and associated predictive analytics can enhance the precision of public health by providing comprehensive insights into disease burden, factors affecting intervention implementation, and outcome measures across various dimensions such as person, place, and time.

MORE PRECISION ASSESSMENT

- **Place**. The use of big data sources could allow a more in-depth analysis of disease burden and implementation gaps and disparities in health-care systems and population subgroups. For example, using small-area analysis might uncover pockets of disparities in the implementation of health interventions that are often masked in the analysis performed on areas such as counties or states.
- **Person**. Similarly, in characterizing gaps and disparities in implementation and outcomes, personal characteristics of patients, providers, and policymakers can be further refined beyond the use of traditional indicators such as age, gender, and race/ethnicity. Genomic and other biomarkers can stratify disease outcomes and susceptibility into subgroups that reflect the underlying disease heterogeneity and potential response to different types of interventions.
- **Time**. Big data may also improve precision through the analysis of repeated measurements of the same variables

[1] “Can Predictive Analytics Drive Implementation Research to Improve Population Health?” Centers for Disease Control and Prevention (CDC), April 9, 2024. Available online. URL: https://blogs.cdc.gov/genomics/2019/05/28/can-predictive-analytics. Accessed September 28, 2024.

over time. The use of personal devices such as sensors, smartphones, and other digital devices can provide measurements of variability over time for various health indicators such as nutrition, physical activity, and blood pressure.

MORE PRECISION IMPLEMENTATION

- **Place**. Implementation studies evaluate the delivery of interventions in real-world contexts of health-care delivery systems and communities. They aim to address the specific needs of different populations effectively.
- **Person**. To reach subpopulations with unique health conditions, targeted intervention strategies will be needed. For example, a decision support tool was recently developed using a machine-learning algorithm based on structured and unstructured data to help identify people with probable familial hypercholesterolemia within electronic health records, large-scale laboratories, and claims databases.
- **Time**. Smartphone apps can use big data to allow real-world collection and analysis over time for many evidence-based interventions (e.g., testing of adherence to medication use and longer-term measuring of outcomes over time). Apps could serve as a microcosm of a learning system that collects data on person, place, and time and uses the patterns detected to adjust an intervention based on its overall pattern of use and effectiveness.

THE ROLE AND CHALLENGES OF PREDICTIVE ANALYTICS

Machine learning and predictive analytic tools are increasingly used in health care and population health settings to make sense of a large amount of data, both for assessment and implementation purposes. In principle, predictive analytics can provide novel approaches to analyzing disease prediction and forecasting models and pinpointing key barriers and facilitators to the delivery of proven effective interventions.

Despite the potential, numerous challenges, such as data inaccuracy, missing information, and selective measurement, must be addressed to ensure the reliability of predictive models.

For precision public health to succeed, further advances in predictive analytics and practical tools for data integration and visualization are needed.[2]

[2] "Can Big Data Science Deliver Precision Public Health?" Centers for Disease Control and Prevention (CDC), April 9, 2024. Available online. URL: https://blogs.cdc.gov/genomics/2019/07/23/can-big-data-science. Accessed September 28, 2024.

Chapter 25 | **Genetic Conditions in Specific Populations**

Chapter Contents

Section 25.1 | Sickle Cell Disease in African and Global Populations

WHAT IS SICKLE CELL DISEASE?

Sickle cell disease (SCD) is a group of inherited red blood cell disorders. Red blood cells contain hemoglobin, a protein that carries oxygen. Healthy red blood cells are round, and they move through small blood vessels to carry oxygen to all parts of the body.

In someone who has SCD, the hemoglobin is abnormal, which causes the red blood cells to become hard and sticky and look like a C-shaped farm tool called a "sickle." The sickle cells die early, which causes a constant shortage of red blood cells. Also, when they travel through small blood vessels, sickle cells get stuck and clog the blood flow. This can cause pain and other serious complications, such as infection, acute chest syndrome, and stroke.

CAUSES OF SICKLE CELL DISEASE

Sickle cell disease is a genetic condition that is present at birth. It is inherited when a child receives two genes—one from each parent—that code for abnormal hemoglobin.[1]

DATA AND STATISTICS ON SICKLE CELL DISEASE

Prevalence of Sickle Cell Disease

WORLDWIDE

Sickle cell disease affects millions of people throughout the world and is particularly common among those whose ancestors came from parts of the world where malaria is or was common:

- Sub-Saharan Africa
- Spanish-speaking regions in the Western Hemisphere (South America, the Caribbean, and Central America)
- Saudi Arabia
- India
- Mediterranean countries such as Turkey, Greece, and Italy

[1] "About Sickle Cell Disease," Centers for Disease Control and Prevention (CDC), September 19, 2024. Available online. URL: www.cdc.gov/sickle-cell/about/index.html. Accessed September 28, 2024.

UNITED STATES

The exact number of people living with SCD in the United States is unknown.

- Two studies published in 2010 estimated that SCD affects approximately 100,000 people in the United States.
- More than 90 percent of people in the United States with SCD are non-Hispanic Black or African American (Black), and an estimated 3–9 percent are Hispanic or Latino.
- SCD occurs in about 1 out of every 365 Black or African-American births and about 1 out of every 16,300 Hispanic-American births.
- About 1 in 13 Black or African-American babies is born with sickle cell trait (SCT; inheritance of a sickle cell gene from only one parent).

Complications and Mortality of Sickle Cell Disease

In people with SCD, red blood cells become rigid and deform into a crescent or sickle shape. The sickled cells die early and often become lodged in small blood vessels, restricting blood flow, which can lead to serious health problems throughout the body.

SCD-associated complications include:

- anemia
- acute and chronic pain
- infections
- pneumonia and acute chest syndrome
- stroke
- kidney, liver, and heart disease

The estimated life expectancy of those with SCD in the United States is more than 20 years shorter than the average expected. Quality-adjusted life expectancy is more than 30 years shorter.

Health-Care Access for Sickle Cell Disease

Despite their extensive health-care needs, many people with SCD have difficulty accessing appropriate care and report feeling stigmatized and having their symptoms dismissed when they do seek care.

In 2014, an expert panel convened by the National Institutes of Health's National Heart, Lung, and Blood Institute (NHLBI) developed recommendations to prevent or reduce complications of SCD. Two of the recommendations were specific to children and adolescents with sickle cell anemia (SCA; the type of SCD that is typically most severe):

- Given that SCA is a common cause of childhood stroke, the panel recommended that children and adolescents aged 2–16 years with SCA be screened annually with transcranial Doppler (TCD) ultrasound to identify those at increased risk for stroke.
- The panel also recommended that children and adolescents aged nine months or older with SCA be offered treatment with hydroxyurea, a medication that has been shown to prevent or reduce severe pain episodes, acute chest syndrome, and other SCA-associated complications and to increase patient survival.

A Centers for Disease Control and Prevention (CDC) study of children and adolescents enrolled in Medicaid found that in 2019 less than half of children and adolescents received the recommended stroke screening.

- Additionally, less than half of children aged 2–9 used hydroxyurea, and approximately one-half of those aged 10–16 used it.
- These findings highlight the ongoing gaps in health care for people with SCD and speak to the urgent need to address barriers to care.[2]

[2] "Data and Statistics on Sickle Cell Disease," Centers for Disease Control and Prevention (CDC), May 15, 2024. Available online. URL: www.cdc.gov/sickle-cell/data/index.html. Accessed September 28, 2024.

Section 25.2 | Cystic Fibrosis in Caucasian Populations

WHAT IS CYSTIC FIBROSIS?

Cystic fibrosis (CF) is a genetic condition that affects a protein in the body. People who have CF have a faulty protein that affects the body's cells, its tissues, and the glands that make mucus and sweat. Normal mucus is slippery and protects the airways, digestive tract, and other organs and tissues. CF causes mucus to become thick and sticky. As mucus builds up, it can cause blockages, damage, or infections in affected organs.

ADVANCES IN SURVIVAL

Cystic fibrosis used to cause death in childhood. Survival has improved because of medical discoveries and advances in newborn screening, medicines, nutrition, and lung transplants. Nearly 40,000 children and adults in the United States and more than 100,000 worldwide are now living with CF. Children born between 2018 and 2022 who have CF are expected to live an average of 56 years. On average, half of babies born in 2021 with CF are expected to reach the age of 65 or older.

SYMPTOMS AND COMPLICATIONS OF CYSTIC FIBROSIS

Some people who have CF have few or no symptoms, while others experience severe symptoms or life-threatening complications. The most serious and common complications of CF are problems with the lungs, including frequent pulmonary or respiratory exacerbations, typically caused by serious lung infections.

Your health-care provider will recommend treatments to improve lung function and prevent or manage complications. Treatment can improve your quality of life and help you live longer.

HOW CYSTIC FIBROSIS AFFECTS YOUR BREATHING

Having a mutation in the *CFTR* gene causes a protein in the body, also called "*CFTR*," to work improperly. This affects how the body makes mucus and sweat. With CF, mucus can be thick and sticky.

This thick mucus can clog up the lungs and airways and make breathing difficult. Bacteria can also grow more easily, which is why lung infections become so common. Difficulties with clearing out mucus in the airways can lead to damage and widening of the airways. This condition is called "bronchiectasis."[1]

CYSTIC FIBROSIS AND INFECTION

Cystic fibrosis is the most frequent hereditary disease in Caucasian populations; chronic microbial colonization of the large airways, leading to exacerbations of pulmonary infection, is the major cause of illness and death in CF patients. Typical CF pathogens include *Staphylococcus aureus*, *Pseudomonas aeruginosa*, *Haemophilus influenzae*, and *Burkholderia cepacia* complex; other species, such as *Stenotrophomonas maltophilia*, *Alcaligenes* (*Achromobacter*) *xylosoxidans*, *Burkholderia gladioli*, and *Ralstonia pickettii*, have been recovered from sputum cultures of CF patients as well. Recently, we showed that a number of unusual bacterial species are also occasionally isolated from CF patients. Infection with mucoid *P. aeruginosa* and members of the *B. cepacia* complex is associated with increased illness and death in CF patients, but the clinical importance of infection with these other species is less clear.

THE GENUS *RALSTONIA*

The genus *Ralstonia* was proposed in 1995. Since its creation, the taxonomy of the genus has expanded to include 11 species, which are:

- *Ralstonia pickettii*
- *Ralstonia solanacearum*
- *Ralstonia eutropha*
- *Ralstonia gilardii*
- *Ralstonia paucula*
- *Ralstonia basilensis*
- *Ralstonia oxalatica*
- *Ralstonia mannitolilytica*

[1] "What Is Cystic Fibrosis?" National Heart, Lung, and Blood Institute (NHLBI), November 21, 2023. Available online. URL: www.nhlbi.nih.gov/health/cystic-fibrosis. Accessed September 28, 2024.

- *Ralstonia taiwanensis*
- *Ralstonia campinensis*
- *Ralstonia metallidurans*

Ralstonia spp. are isolated from a wide variety of ecological niches, including plants and soils contaminated with heavy metals. *R. pickettii* has been associated with nosocomial outbreaks caused by contaminated solutions used for patient care and with pseudoepidemics caused by contaminated solutions in the diagnostic laboratory. *R. paucula* and *R. gilardii* have only sporadically been isolated from human clinical samples, including cerebrospinal fluid, bone marrow, wounds, and the respiratory tract. A complete assessment of the frequency of human infection due to *Ralstonia* species is confounded by the difficulty in accurate species identification by using standard microbiologic techniques. Indeed, these species are frequently misidentified as *Pseudomonas fluorescens* or *Burkholderia cepacia* complex.[2]

Section 25.3 | Thalassemia Prevalence in Mediterranean and Southern Asian Populations

THALASSEMIA: AN INHERITED BLOOD DISORDER

A thalassemia is a group of inherited blood diseases that affect a person's ability to produce hemoglobin, resulting in anemia. Hemoglobin is a protein in red blood cells that carries oxygen and nutrients to cells in the body. About 100,000 babies worldwide are born each year with severe forms of thalassemia. Thalassemia occurs most frequently in people of Italian, Greek, Middle Eastern, Southern Asian, and African ancestry.

[2] "Infection by *Ralstonia* Species in Cystic Fibrosis Patients: Identification of *R. pickettii* and *R. mannitolilytica* by Polymerase Chain Reaction," Centers for Disease Control and Prevention (CDC), July 2002. Available online. URL: wwwnc.cdc.gov/eid/article/8/7/01-0472_article. Accessed September 28, 2024.

TYPES OF THALASSEMIA

The two main types of thalassemia are called "alpha" and "beta," depending on which part of an oxygen-carrying protein in the red blood cells is lacking. Both types of thalassemia are inherited in the same manner. The disease is passed to children by parents who carry the mutated thalassemia gene. A child who inherits one mutated gene is a carrier, which is sometimes called the "thalassemia trait." Most carriers lead completely normal, healthy lives.

A child who inherits two thalassemia trait genes—one from each parent—will have the disease. A child of two carriers has a 25 percent chance of receiving two trait genes and developing the disease and a 50 percent chance of being a thalassemia trait carrier.

Most people with alpha thalassemia have milder forms of the disease, with varying degrees of anemia. The most severe form of alpha thalassemia, which affects mainly people of Southeast Asian, Chinese, and Filipino ancestry, results in fetal or newborn death.

A child who inherits two copies of the mutated gene for beta thalassemia will have beta thalassemia disease. The child can have a mild form of the disease, known as "thalassemia intermedia," which causes milder anemia that rarely requires transfusions.

THALASSEMIA MAJOR

The more severe form of the disease is thalassemia major, also called "Cooley anemia." It is a serious disease that requires regular blood transfusions and extensive medical care.

Those with thalassemia major usually show symptoms within the first two years of life. They become pale and listless and have poor appetites. They grow slowly and often develop jaundice. Without treatment, the spleen, liver, and heart soon become greatly enlarged. Bones become thin and brittle. Heart failure and infection are the leading causes of death among children with untreated thalassemia major.

The use of frequent blood transfusions and antibiotics has improved the outlook for children with thalassemia major. Frequent transfusions keep their hemoglobin levels near normal and prevent many of the complications of the disease. However, repeated blood transfusions lead to iron overload—a buildup of iron in the body—that can damage the heart, liver, and other organs. Drugs known as "iron chelators" can help rid the body of excess iron, preventing or delaying problems related to iron overload.

Thalassemia has been cured using bone marrow transplants. However, this treatment is possible only for a small minority of patients who have a suitable bone marrow donor. The transplant procedure itself is still risky and can result in death.

ADVANCEMENTS IN GENE THERAPY FOR THALASSEMIA

Scientists are working to develop a gene therapy that may offer a cure for thalassemia. Such a treatment might involve inserting a normal beta-globin gene (the gene that is abnormal in this disease) into the patient's stem cells, the immature bone marrow cells that are the precursors of all other cells in the blood.

Another form of gene therapy could involve using drugs or other methods to reactivate the patient's genes that produce fetal hemoglobin—the form of hemoglobin found in fetuses and newborns. Scientists hope that spurring the production of fetal hemoglobin will compensate for the patient's deficiency of adult hemoglobin.

GENETIC TESTING AND REPRODUCTIVE OPTIONS FOR THALASSEMIA

Blood tests and family genetic studies can show whether a person has thalassemia or is a carrier. If both parents are carriers, they may want to consult with a genetic counselor for help in deciding whether to conceive or whether to have a fetus tested for thalassemia.

Prenatal testing can be done using chorionic villus sampling (CVS) around the 11th week of pregnancy. This involves removing a tiny piece of the placenta. The fetus can also be tested with amniocentesis around the 16th week of pregnancy. In this procedure, a needle is used to take a sample of the fluid surrounding the baby for testing.

Assisted reproductive therapy is also an option for carriers who do not want to risk giving birth to a child with thalassemia. A new technique, preimplantation genetic diagnosis (PGD), used in conjunction with in vitro fertilization, may enable parents who have thalassemia or carry the trait to give birth to healthy babies. Embryos created in vitro are tested for the thalassemia gene before being implanted into the mother, allowing only healthy embryos to be selected.[1]

[1] "About Thalassemia," National Human Genome Research Institute (NHGRI), December 27, 2013. Available online. URL: www.genome.gov/Genetic-Disorders/Thalassemia. Accessed September 28, 2024.

Chapter 26 | **Personalized Medicine and Diverse Population Studies**

WHAT IS PERSONALIZED MEDICINE?

Personalized medicine is an emerging practice that uses an individual's genetic profile to guide decisions regarding the prevention, diagnosis, and treatment of disease. Knowledge of a patient's genetic profile can help doctors select the proper medication or therapy and administer it at the proper dose or regimen. Personalized medicine is being advanced through data from the Human Genome Project.[1]

LARGE-SCALE POPULATION STUDIES AS A PATH TO PERSONALIZED MEDICINE

Scientific evaluation of new gene discoveries has been aided by the launch of large-scale epidemiologic and clinical collaborative global studies. In a recent commentary, Muin J. Khoury and Marta Gwinn (Office of Genomics and Precision Public Health, Centers for Disease Control and Prevention [CDC]) argue that these studies can provide an evidentiary path to personalized medicine—but only if they are done in diverse populations and integrate rare and common genetic risk factors with measurements of changing environments and health indices over time.

[1] "Personalized Medicine," National Human Genome Research Institute (NHGRI), September 27, 2024. Available online. URL: www.genome.gov/genetics-glossary/Personalized-Medicine. Accessed September 28, 2024.

INTEGRATING RARE AND COMMON GENETIC RISK FACTORS INTO A GENETIC RISK SCORE

The National Institutes of Health's (NIH) Genetic Testing Registry (GTR), which collects information on tests in clinical use, currently includes tests for more than 18,000 disorders; these include relatively rare heritable diseases such as cystic fibrosis (CF) and sickle cell disease (SCD), along with many others. Genetic risk factors for common diseases include thousands of variants identified by genome-wide association studies; however, their individual effects on risk are too small to have much predictive value, leading some researchers to propose polygenic risk scores. Most data used to construct polygenic risk scores come from people of European descent. These scores may perform poorly when used in other populations, especially in racial and ethnic minorities, where their use could produce erroneous risk estimates and exacerbate health disparities. Studies that incorporate sequencing are also revealing the role of rare variants with substantial effects in carriers (e.g., *BRCA1* and *BRCA2* in breast and ovarian cancer). Risk scores that integrate information on common and rare variants will produce more precise individual estimates of genetic risk than those based on either alone.

INTEGRATING GENETIC WITH ENVIRONMENTAL RISK FACTORS

When McCarthy, executive director of Human Genetics at Genentech, South San Francisco, California, USA and Birney, deputy director-general of the European Molecular Biology Laboratory, Cambridge, UK state, "there is more to disease risk than genetics," it appears that they are addressing geneticists. They could just as well suggest that epidemiologists look beyond environmental and socioeconomic factors or remind clinicians to look beyond routine laboratory values. Genetic and non-genetic risk factors interact in ways that can often be hard to measure, much less integrate in a way that informs risk estimates. Even for well-characterized factors, such as smoking and exercise, the lifetime effect on disease is difficult to construct using cross-sectional measurements (e.g., the number of steps walked last week). In addition, social determinants of health, such as access to health care, education, and housing, have major effects on disease risk and outcomes. Just as with genetic risk, epidemiologic models based on narrowly selected populations (such as well-off, well-educated volunteers) may not translate accurately to other communities.

INTEGRATING CLINICAL INFORMATION OVER TIME

Gathering clinical measurements over time can improve disease risk estimation. Snapshots of clinical and laboratory measurements may have limited predictive ability, whereas the availability of longitudinal data (e.g., electronic health records and wearable devices) could improve prediction. For example, a recent study modeled 2.1 billion measurements from 92 different laboratory tests in 2.8 million adults over a span of 18 years. For 131 chronic conditions and 5,223 drug–test pairs, they assessed test distributions in healthy individuals. Age and sex alone explain less than 10 percent of the test variance in 89 out of 92 tests. However, personalized models based on patients' history explain 60 percent of the variance for 17 tests and over 36 percent of the variance for half of the tests. This proof-of-concept study points to the potential utility of systematic stratification of risk for subsequent disease development.

EMBRACING COMPLEXITY AND AVOIDING ARTIFICIAL CATEGORIZATION OF RISK FACTORS

Most diseases represent a confluence of pathological processes, even in the same person. For example, heart disease may be due to a combination of processes such as glucose metabolism, lipid disorders, high blood pressure (HBP), and inflammation. The precise combination will be different from one person to another and across each person's lifetime. McCarthy and Birney recommend that when several processes contribute to disease, it makes sense to track each process over time rather than collapse information into arbitrary disease or risk categories.

It is perhaps not surprising that the path to personalized medicine should start with large-scale longitudinal population studies. Nevertheless, these studies will take years, if not decades, to complete, and they are very expensive and complex. Furthermore, they can have methodological pitfalls in the selection of participants, measurement of risk factors and outcomes, data standardization and sharing, complex analyses, and causal inference. In the meantime, adding implementation science to these studies can inform how best to deploy interventions that can save lives and reduce health disparities.[2]

[2] "Large-Scale Population Studies as a Path to Personalized Medicine: Easier Said than Done!" Centers for Disease Control and Prevention (CDC), September 22, 2021. Available online. URL: https://blogs.cdc.gov/genomics/2021/09/22/how-large-scale. Accessed September 28, 2024.

Chapter 27 | Pharmacogenomics: Personalized Drug Responses

Pharmacogenomics is an important example of the field of precision medicine, which aims to tailor medical treatment to each person or to a group of people. Pharmacogenomics looks at how your DNA (deoxyribonucleic acid) affects the way you respond to drugs. In some cases, your DNA can affect whether you have a bad reaction to a drug or whether a drug helps you or has no effect. Pharmacogenomics can improve your health by helping you know ahead of time whether a drug is likely to benefit you and be safe for you to take. Knowing this information can help your health-care provider find medicine that will work best for you.

HOW IT WORKS

Drugs interact with your body in many ways, depending both on how you take the drug and where the drug acts in your body. After you take a drug, your body needs to break it down and get it to the intended area. Your DNA can affect multiple steps in this process to influence how you respond to the drug. Some examples of these interactions are described here.

Drug Receptors

Some drugs need to attach to proteins on the surface of cells, called "receptors," in order to work properly. Your DNA determines what type of receptors you have, and how many, which can affect your response to the drug. You might need a higher or lower amount of the drug than most people, or you might need an entirely different drug.

EXAMPLE: BREAST CANCER AND T-DM1

Some breast cancers make too much HER2, a receptor, and this extra HER2 helps the cancer develop and spread. The drug T-DM1 can be used to treat this type of breast cancer and works by attaching to HER2 on cancerous cells and killing them. If you have breast cancer, your health-care provider may test a sample of your tumor to determine if T-DM1 is the right treatment for you. If your tumor has a high amount of HER2 (HER2-positive), your health-care provider may prescribe T-DM1. If your tumor does not have enough HER2 (HER2-negative), T-DM1 will not work for you.

Drug Uptake

Some drugs need to be actively taken into the tissues and cells in which they act. Your DNA can affect uptake of certain drugs. Decreased uptake can mean that the drug does not work as well and can cause it to build up in other parts of your body, which can cause problems. Your DNA can also affect how quickly some drugs are removed from the cells in which they act. If drugs are removed from the cells too quickly, they might not have time to act.

EXAMPLE: STATINS AND MUSCLE PROBLEMS

Statins are a type of drug that act in the liver to help lower cholesterol. In order for statins to work correctly, they must first be taken into the liver. Statins are transported into the liver by a protein made by the *SLCO1B1* gene. Some people have a specific change in this gene that causes less of a statin called "simvastatin" to be taken into the liver. When taken at high doses, simvastatin can build up in the blood, causing muscle problems, including weakness and pain. Before prescribing simvastatin, your health-care provider may recommend genetic testing for the *SLCO1B1* gene to check if simvastatin is the best statin for you or to determine what dose would work best.

Drug Breakdown

Your DNA can affect how quickly your body breaks down a drug. If you break the drug down more quickly than most people, your body gets rid of the drug faster, and you might need more of the drug or a different drug. If your body breaks the drug down more slowly, you might need less of the drug.

EXAMPLE: DEPRESSION AND AMITRIPTYLINE

The breakdown of the antidepressant drug amitriptyline is influenced by two genes called "*CYP2D6*" and "*CYP2C19*." If your health-care provider prescribes amitriptyline, they might recommend genetic testing for the *CYP2D6* and *CYP2C19* genes to help decide what dose of the drug you need. If you break down amitriptyline too fast, you will need a higher dose for it to work, or you may need to use a different drug. If you break down amitriptyline very slowly, you will need to take a smaller dose or will need to take a different drug to avoid a bad reaction.

Targeted Drug Development

Pharmacogenomic approaches to drug development target the underlying problem rather than just treating symptoms. Some diseases are caused by specific changes (mutations) in a gene. The same gene can have different types of changes, which have different effects. Some genetic changes may result in a protein that does not work correctly, while others may mean that the protein is not made at all. Drugs can be created based on how the genetic change affects the protein, and these drugs will only work for a specific type of genetic change.

EXAMPLE: CYSTIC FIBROSIS AND IVACAFTOR

Cystic fibrosis is caused by genetic changes in the *CFTR* gene that affect the CFTR protein. The CFTR protein forms a channel, which acts as a passageway to move particles across the cells in your body. For most people, the protein is made correctly, and the channel can open and close. Some genetic changes that cause cystic fibrosis result in a channel that is closed. The drug ivacaftor acts on this type of genetic change by forcing the channel open. Ivacaftor would not be expected to work for people with cystic fibrosis whose genetic change causes the channel not to be made at all.

WHAT IT MEANS FOR YOU

While pharmacogenomic testing is currently used for only a few drugs, the field is growing very quickly. Improved understanding of how pharmacogenomics can protect your health and improve your treatment will be increasingly important. Talk to your health-care provider about what pharmacogenomics might mean for your health.[1]

[1] "Pharmacogenomics," Centers for Disease Control and Prevention (CDC), May 15, 2024. Available online. URL: www.cdc.gov/genomics-and-health/about/pharmacogenetics.html. Accessed September 28, 2024.

Part 5 | Prevalence and Patterns of Common Conditions across Demographic Groups

Chapter 28 | Cardiovascular Disease and Demographics

Chapter Contents

Section 28.1 | Poverty, Hypertension, and Cardiovascular Disease in Racial and Ethnic Groups

Cardiovascular disease (CVD) is the leading cause of death in the United States. Certain demographic characteristics are associated with disparities in CVD and its risk factors, which may interact with specific social determinants of health (SDOH).

RACIAL AND ETHNIC DISPARITIES IN HYPERTENSION CONTROL

In a 2021 study that used National Health and Nutrition Examination Survey (NHANES) data, non-Hispanic Black and Hispanic participants had a significantly lower prevalence of blood pressure control (39% and 40%, respectively) than their non-Hispanic white counterparts (49%). Findings on the prevalence of awareness and treatment of hypertension among these groups were discordant with findings on the prevalence of hypertension. Although the prevalence of hypertension awareness and treatment was similar among non-Hispanic Black and non-Hispanic white participants, the prevalence of hypertension was significantly higher among non-Hispanic Black participants (45.5% vs. 31.4%). Conversely, the prevalence of hypertension awareness and treatment was lower among Hispanic participants than non-Hispanic white participants, but the two groups had a similar prevalence of hypertension. The higher prevalence of hypertension observed among non-Hispanic Black participants may disproportionately increase their risk of CVD.

SOCIAL DETERMINANTS OF HEALTH AND CARDIOVASCULAR DISEASE

Some demographic characteristics, such as age and sex, are well known to increase the risk for CVD. Less well-described are the effects of SDOH (e.g., income, educational attainment, employment status, psychosocial factors including racism, and environmental factors)—all of which are key indicators of health disparities. U.S. studies have shown that people in higher income groups experience lower rates of CVD events than people in low-income groups. Educational attainment was found to have an inverse relationship with the prevalence of CVD morbidity.

The intersection of SDOH and hypertension can create health disparities and affect the prevalence of CVD morbidity. Specific SDOH may interact with hypertension to have a combined effect that leads to an excess burden of CVD morbidity. Additionally, SDOH may also negatively affect specific populations and lead to hypertension. Intersectionality, defined by the National Collaborating Centre for Healthy Public Policy, is a useful concept to address these risk factors for CVD.

POVERTY, STRESSORS, AND CARDIOVASCULAR HEALTH DISPARITIES

People experiencing poverty and those who are financially and medically underresourced may be more likely than their wealthier and better-resourced counterparts to be exposed to psychosocial and socioeconomic stressors, discrimination, and racism, which can exacerbate the lack of hypertension control and increase CVD disparities.

This study compiled 19 years of NHANES data and analyzed the combined exposure of poverty and hypertension on the prevalence of CVD that exceeded the expected prevalence of CVD among Hispanic, non-Hispanic Black, and non-Hispanic white participants. One key finding is that poverty level was independently associated with an increased risk for diagnosed CVD morbidity among all three racial and ethnic groups studied. In addition, low educational attainment (i.e., less than college education) was found to be a strong predictor of CVD among non-Hispanic white participants but not among non-Hispanic Black and Hispanic participants. Previous studies support that low educational attainment may be associated with CVD because of behavioral characteristics, such as smoking, lack of physical activity, and obesity, in addition to other SDOH.

HEALTH DISPARITIES AMONG RACIAL AND ETHNIC GROUPS

It is well established that certain populations experience health disparities and are disproportionately affected by CVD and hypertension.

Additionally, a working poor segment of the U.S. population meets the poverty–income ratio or poverty threshold; they often do not have health insurance and are not eligible for federal assistance programs such as the Supplemental Nutrition Assistance Program. Our results show that one key SDOH, poverty, may interact with hypertension to influence diagnosed CVD morbidity disproportionately among certain groups. This result is exemplified by the larger additive interaction of poverty and hypertension among non-Hispanic Black and Hispanic people compared with non-Hispanic white people. Although not statistically significant, the larger additive interaction among non-Hispanic Black and Hispanic people is noteworthy and clinically relevant. This excess burden of diagnosed CVD morbidity among non-Hispanic Black and Hispanic people, resulting from the intersection of poverty, race and ethnicity, and hypertension, may lead to health disparities. Similar results were found by a study that analyzed the risk of hypertension by income, racial and ethnic composition, and geographic location. The study showed that non-Hispanic white participants with higher incomes had significantly lower odds of hypertension than non-Hispanic Black participants with low incomes (24% vs. 52%).

ADDRESSING SOCIAL DETERMINANTS OF HEALTH IN PUBLIC HEALTH INTERVENTIONS

Observable SDOH, such as poverty, are influenced by numerous factors at multiple levels. SDOH include all aspects of life, such as the places where people live, work, and play. If the public health and medical communities are to reduce the equity gap in CVD among certain populations (i.e., race and ethnicity or low income), then the convergence of upstream psychosocial and socioeconomic stressors, such as poverty, depression, job stress, financial stress, segregated neighborhoods, and neighborhood poverty level, should be considered. Furthermore, efforts designed to reduce disparities in the prevalence of diagnosed CVD morbidity may need to address the convergence of these multilevel risk factors. These SDOH are modifiable. In a scenario where the negative effects of an SDOH can be alleviated, the prevalence would decrease not only by the SDOH's independent effect but also by its excess morbidity with hypertension. By analyzing the additive interaction and assessing the excess morbidity, public health and policy officials can intuitively see the ramifications of any potential intervention that disrupts the interaction. These ramifications can be seen intuitively because the assessment of an additive interaction is performed in an absolute manner rather than by interpreting the results of multiplicative interactions, which are relative to one another.

THE ROLE OF DISCRIMINATION AND RACISM

Other factors and stressors—such as discrimination and racism—may be considered. A study that examined the relationship between blood pressure and self-reported racial discrimination and responses to unfair treatment found a significant association between hypertension and racial discrimination. Characteristics historically linked to racism, discrimination, and exclusion are factors that may be incorporated into interventions to address inequities in the prevalence of CVD morbidity. Public health interventions that also address racism may need to be considered to meet the diverse needs of populations who are affected by racism and are medically underserved. The consequences of centuries of racism are pervasive, deeply embedded in society, and have a negative effect on racial and ethnic minority populations. The potentially strong repercussions of discrimination, racism, and health-care disparities resulting from treatment or implicit bias (i.e., people receiving inadequate treatment of hypertension because of language barriers or their race or ethnicity) are important factors that could be considered. Racism and discrimination may play a role as a stressor and determinant of health that detrimentally affects blood pressure and heart health for non-Hispanic Black people in the United States.

POLICY RECOMMENDATIONS AND FUTURE DIRECTIONS

The Surgeon General's Call to Action on Hypertension describes the historical consequences of racial discrimination, identifies SDOH as the "third arm of risk," and expresses the need to equitably distribute human, technical, and financial resources to address these factors. Furthermore, in its 2010 report, *A Population-Based Policy and Systems Change Approach to Prevent and Control Hypertension*, the Institute of Medicine suggests integrating hypertension prevention and control interventions into the policies and programs of public health practices in ways that support healthy eating, active living, and obesity, as well as focusing on populations that are most likely to be affected by hypertension. In addition, population-based policy interventions focusing on systems-level improvements in SDOH, such as poverty, food insecurity, low educational attainment, and language barriers, may be considered when seeking ways to address disparities in the prevalence of CVD morbidity.[1]

Section 28.2 | **Contributing Factors to Heart Disease**

RISK FACTORS FOR HEART DISEASE

Several health conditions, lifestyle choices, age, and family history can increase the risk for heart disease. These are referred to as "risk factors." About half of all Americans (47%) have at least one of three key risk factors for heart disease:

- high blood pressure (HBP)
- high cholesterol
- smoking

Some risk factors for heart disease, such as age or family history, cannot be controlled. However, steps can be taken to lower the risk by changing the factors that can be controlled.

CONDITIONS THAT CAN INCREASE RISK

High Blood Pressure

High blood pressure is a major risk factor for heart disease. It is a medical condition that occurs when the pressure of the blood in

[1] "Excess Burden of Poverty and Hypertension, by Race and Ethnicity, on the Prevalence of Cardiovascular Disease," Centers for Disease Control and Prevention (CDC), November 22, 2023. Available online. URL: www.cdc.gov/pcd/issues/2023/23_0065.htm. Accessed September 30, 2024.

the arteries and other blood vessels is too high. If not controlled, HBP can affect the heart and other major organs, including the kidneys and brain.

HBP is often called a "silent killer" because it usually has no symptoms. The only way to know whether you have HBP is to measure it. Blood pressure can be lowered with lifestyle changes or medication to reduce the risk for heart disease and heart attack.

Unhealthy Blood Cholesterol Levels

Cholesterol is a waxy, fat-like substance made by the liver or found in certain foods. The liver makes enough cholesterol for the body's needs, but excess cholesterol from food can build up in the walls of the arteries, including those of the heart. This leads to the narrowing of the arteries and can decrease blood flow to the heart, brain, kidneys, and other parts of the body.

There are two main types of blood cholesterol:

1. **LDL (low-density lipoprotein) cholesterol.** Considered "bad" cholesterol because it can cause plaque buildup in the arteries.
2. **HDL (high-density lipoprotein) cholesterol.** Considered "good" cholesterol because higher levels provide some protection against heart disease.

High blood cholesterol usually has no signs or symptoms. The only way to know whether you have high cholesterol is to get it checked through a blood test called a "lipid profile."

Diabetes Mellitus

The body needs glucose (sugar) for energy. Insulin is a hormone made in the pancreas that helps move glucose from the food consumed into the body's cells for energy. If diabetes is present, the body does not make enough insulin, cannot use its own insulin effectively, or both.

Diabetes causes sugar to build up in the blood, increasing the risk of death from heart disease compared to individuals without diabetes. It is important to talk with a doctor about ways to prevent or manage diabetes and control other risk factors.

Obesity

Obesity is defined as excess body fat and is linked to higher levels of "bad" cholesterol and triglycerides and lower levels of "good" cholesterol. It can lead to HBP, diabetes, and heart disease. Consulting with a health-care team about a plan to reduce weight to a healthy level is recommended.

LIFESTYLE CHOICES THAT CAN INCREASE RISK

Unhealthy Diet

Eating a diet high in saturated fats, *trans* fats, and cholesterol is linked to heart disease and related conditions such as atherosclerosis. Additionally, excessive salt (sodium) intake can raise blood pressure.

Physical Inactivity

Not getting enough physical activity can lead to heart disease and increase the chances of developing other medical conditions that are risk factors, including obesity, HBP, high cholesterol, and diabetes. Regular physical activity can lower the risk for heart disease.

Excessive Alcohol Consumption

Drinking too much alcohol can raise blood pressure levels and the risk for heart disease. It also increases triglyceride levels, which can further increase the risk for heart disease. Women should consume no more than one drink per day, and men should consume no more than two drinks per day.

Tobacco Use

Smoking cigarettes increases the risk for heart disease and heart attack. It can damage the heart and blood vessels, leading to conditions such as atherosclerosis and heart attack. Nicotine raises blood pressure, and carbon monoxide from cigarette smoke reduces the amount of oxygen that blood can carry. Exposure to secondhand smoke can also increase the risk for heart disease, even for nonsmokers.

OTHER FACTORS THAT CAN INCREASE RISK

Genetics and Family History

Heredity plays a role in passing traits from one generation to another through genes. Genetic factors likely contribute to HBP, heart disease, and other related conditions. However, individuals with a family history of heart disease may also share common environments and other factors that increase their risk. The risk for heart disease can further increase when heredity combines with unhealthy lifestyle choices, such as smoking and an unhealthy diet.

Age and Sex

Heart disease is the number one killer of both men and women. While it can occur at any age, the risk increases with age.

Race and Ethnicity

Heart disease and stroke can affect anyone, but certain groups are more likely to have conditions that increase their risk for cardiovascular disease. Heart disease is the leading cause of death for most racial and ethnic groups in the United States, including African Americans, American Indians and Alaska Natives, and white people. For Asian-American, Pacific-Islander, and Hispanic people, heart disease is second only to cancer.[1]

Section 28.3 | Global Approaches to Preventing and Managing Cardiovascular Diseases

Cardiovascular disease (CVD), a group of disorders of the heart and blood vessels that includes coronary heart disease, stroke, congestive heart failure, and other conditions, is the leading cause of death worldwide and a major contributor to disability. In 2020, an estimated 523 million people had some form of CVD, and

[1] "Heart Disease Risk Factors," Centers for Disease Control and Prevention (CDC), May 15, 2024. Available online. URL: www.cdc.gov/heart-disease/risk-factors/index.html. Accessed September 30, 2024.

approximately 19 million deaths were attributable to CVD; this represents approximately 32 percent of all global deaths and is an absolute increase of 18.7 percent from 2010.

GLOBAL TRENDS IN CARDIOVASCULAR DISEASE BURDEN

Global trends for disability-adjusted life years for CVD and the CVD burden attributable to modifiable risk factors have also continued to increase steadily since 1990. In the United States, nearly half of adults (approximately 127 million) had one or more CVD conditions. Provisional mortality data for 2021 indicate that even during the coronavirus 2019 (COVID-19) pandemic, heart disease and stroke remained the first and the fifth leading causes of death in the United States, respectively.

Despite advancements in the management of CVD and other health outcomes worldwide, minority, disadvantaged, and underserved populations continue to experience significant health disparities, with these disparities exacerbated during the COVID-19 pandemic.

ADVANCES IN THE PREVENTION AND MANAGEMENT OF CARDIOVASCULAR DISEASE

In recent years, researchers and public health programs and practices have focused on preventing, managing, and controlling traditional CVD risk factors by instituting timely intervention programs, identifying social determinants of health (SDOH), examining disparities in CVD risks, assessing the COVID-19 pandemic's effect on CVD risks, and implementing collective efforts through community-based approaches to achieve population-level improvements in cardiovascular health.

MAJOR CONTRIBUTORS TO CARDIOVASCULAR DISEASE-RELATED MORTALITY

The greatest contributors to CVD-related years of life lost globally are:

- tobacco exposure
- hypertension
- high body mass index (BMI)
- high fasting plasma glucose

Tobacco exposure, including cigarette smoking, secondhand smoke, and use of smokeless tobacco, contributed to 8.7 million deaths worldwide in 2019, one-third of which were due to CVD.

Hypertension affects more than 4 billion people worldwide, representing a near doubling in the absolute prevalence of hypertension since 1990. In the United States, nearly half of adults (47%) have hypertension, but only about one in four (24%) have their condition under control.

High BMI continues to increase globally, with significant effects on death, disability, and quality of life. The prevalence of obesity has increased worldwide in the past 50 years, reaching pandemic levels. Obesity represents a major health challenge because it substantially increases the risk of diseases such as hypertension, myocardial infarction, stroke, type 2 diabetes, and dementia, thereby contributing to a decline in both quality of life and life expectancy.

Furthermore, global increases in high fasting plasma glucose and its sequelae, type 2 diabetes, have mirrored the increases seen in BMI over the past three decades.

Other risks that contribute to increased CVD burden and disparities in cardiovascular morbidity and mortality are as follows:

- behavioral risks
  - unhealthy diet
  - physical inactivity
  - inadequate sleep
  - excessive alcohol use
- environmental risks
  - air pollution
  - extreme temperatures
- social risks
  - house insecurity
  - food insecurity

CARDIOVASCULAR DISEASE AS INDICATORS OF GLOBAL HEALTH DISPARITIES

Cardiovascular disease and its related risk factors are increasingly recognized as growing indicators of global health disparities. Globally, differences in morbidity and mortality from

CVD exist among high, middle, and low-income countries and across ethnic groups. In the United States, disparities in CVD morbidity, mortality, and risk factors have persisted for decades, with concerning stagnation and significant upward trends since the early 2000s.

Disparities are largely influenced by demographic, socioeconomic, and environmental factors. For example, African-American and American Indian adults experience a higher burden of cardiovascular risk factors and CVD compared with non-Hispanic white adults. Unfortunately, structural racism remains a significant cause of poor cardiovascular health, restricting racial and ethnic minority populations from opportunities to live healthier lives in healthier neighborhoods and from access to quality education and health care.

STRATEGIES FOR REDUCING CARDIOVASCULAR DISEASE RISK AND ADVANCING HEALTH EQUITY

Decreasing CVD risk requires strong, diverse collaborations and the implementation of innovative approaches that aim to eliminate health disparities and advance health equity in diverse environments and contexts. Eliminating health disparities and advancing health equity should be core components in all research, evaluation, and programmatic activities and require a focus on SDOH. Systematically addressing SDOH requires multisectoral commitment and the implementation of evidence-based public policies and actions across all sectors.

Countries that employ multisectoral approaches are better able to identify and address issues around poverty, housing, and others by working collaboratively across sectors, with multisectoral action by governments to achieve health equity.[1]

[1] "Global Responses to Prevent, Manage, and Control Cardiovascular Diseases," Centers for Disease Control and Prevention (CDC), December 8, 2022. Available online. URL: www.cdc.gov/pcd/issues/2022/22_0347.htm. Accessed September 30, 2024.

Chapter 29 | Prevalence and Incidence of Diabetes in the United States

NATIONAL DIABETES STATISTICS REPORT

The National Diabetes Statistics Report provides up-to-date information on the prevalence and incidence of diabetes and prediabetes, risk factors for complications, acute and long-term complications, deaths, and costs.

FAST FACTS ON DIABETES

Diabetes

- **Total**. 38.4 million people have diabetes (11.6% of the U.S. population).
- **Diagnosed**. 29.7 million people, including 29.4 million adults.
- **Undiagnosed**. 8.7 million people (22.8% of adults with diabetes are undiagnosed).

Prediabetes

- **Total**. 97.6 million people aged 18 years or older have prediabetes (38% of the adult U.S. population).
- **65 years or older**. 27.2 million people aged 65 years or older (48.8%) have prediabetes.

PREVALENCE OF BOTH DIAGNOSED AND UNDIAGNOSED DIABETES

Among the U.S. population overall, crude estimates for 2021 were:

- 38.4 million people of all ages—or 11.6 percent of the U.S. population—had diabetes.
- 38.1 million adults aged 18 years or older—or 14.7 percent of all U.S. adults—had diabetes.
- 8.7 million adults aged 18 years or older who met laboratory criteria for diabetes were not aware of or did not report having diabetes (undiagnosed diabetes). This number represents 3.4 percent of all U.S. adults and 22.8 percent of all U.S. adults with diabetes.
- The percentage of adults with diabetes increased with age, reaching 29.2 percent among those aged 65 years or older.

PREVALENCE OF DIAGNOSED DIABETES

Among the U.S. population overall, crude estimates for 2021 were:

- 29.7 million people of all ages—or 8.9 percent of the U.S. population—had been diagnosed with diabetes.
- 352,000 children and adolescents younger than age 20 years—or 35 per 10,000 U.S. youths—had diagnosed diabetes. This includes 304,000 with type 1 diabetes.
- 1.7 million adults aged 20 years or older—or 5.7 percent of all U.S. adults with diagnosed diabetes—reported both having type 1 diabetes and using insulin.
- 3.6 million adults aged 20 years or older—or 12.3 percent of all U.S. adults with diagnosed diabetes—started using insulin within a year of their diagnosis.
- Among U.S. adults aged 18 years or older, age-adjusted data for 2019–2021 indicated the following:
    - For both men and women, the prevalence of diagnosed diabetes was highest among American Indian and Alaska Native adults (13.6%), followed by non-Hispanic Black adults (12.1%), adults of Hispanic origin (11.7%), non-Hispanic Asian

adults (9.1%), and non-Hispanic white adults (6.9%).

- Prevalence varied significantly by education level, which is an indicator of socioeconomic status. Specifically, 13.1 percent of adults with less than a high school education had been diagnosed with diabetes versus 9.1 percent of those with a high school education and 6.9 percent of those with more than a high school education.
- Adults with family income above 500 percent of the federal poverty level had the lowest prevalence, for both men (6.3%) and women (3.9%).
- For both men and women, prevalence was higher among adults living in nonmetropolitan areas compared to those in metropolitan areas.

INCIDENCE OF NEWLY DIAGNOSED DIABETES

Incidence among Adults

Among U.S. adults aged 18 years or older, crude estimates for 2021 were:

- 1.2 million new cases of diabetes—or 5.9 per 1,000 people—were diagnosed.
- Compared to adults aged 18–44 years, incidence rates of diagnosed diabetes were higher among adults aged 45–64 years and those aged 65 years and older.
- Among U.S. adults aged 18 years or older, age-adjusted data for 2019–2021 indicated:
    - Incidence estimates were higher for non-Hispanic Black adults and Hispanic adults than for non-Hispanic white adults and Asian adults.
    - Incidence rates of diagnosed diabetes were higher among those with less than a high school education and those with a high school education only compared to adults with more than a high school education.
    - Incidence was similar among adults living in metropolitan and nonmetropolitan areas.

Incidence among Children and Adolescents

Data from the SEARCH for Diabetes in Youth study indicated that, during 2017–2018, the estimated annual number of newly diagnosed cases in the United States included:

- 18,169 children and adolescents younger than age 20 years with type 1 diabetes
- 5,293 children and adolescents aged 10–19 years with type 2 diabetes

Prevalence of Prediabetes among Adults

- An estimated 97.6 million adults aged 18 years or older had prediabetes in 2021.
- Among U.S. adults aged 18 years or older, crude estimates for 2017–2020 were:
    - 38 percent of all U.S. adults had prediabetes, based on their fasting glucose or A1C level.
    - 19 percent of adults with prediabetes reported being told by a health professional that they had this condition.

RISK FACTORS FOR DIABETES-RELATED COMPLICATIONS

Among U.S. adults aged 18 years or older with diagnosed diabetes, crude estimates for 2017–2020 were:

Smoking

- 22.1 percent were tobacco users based on self-report or levels of serum cotinine.
- 14.6 percent reported current cigarette smoking.
- 36 percent had quit smoking but had a history of smoking at least 100 cigarettes in their lifetime.

Overweight and Obesity

- 89.8 percent were overweight or had obesity, defined as a body mass index (BMI) of 25 kg/m^2 or higher. Specifically:
    - 26.9 percent were overweight (BMI of 25.0–29.9 kg/m^2).
    - 47.1 percent had obesity (BMI of 30.0–39.9 kg/m^2).

- 15.7 percent had extreme obesity (BMI of 40.0 kg/m^2 or higher).

Physical Inactivity

- 31.9 percent were physically inactive, defined as getting less than 10 minutes a week of moderate or vigorous activity in each physical activity category of work, leisure time, and transportation.

A1C

- 47.4 percent had an A1C value of 7.0 percent or higher. Specifically:
  - 22.9 percent had an A1C value of 7.0–7.9 percent.
  - 11.5 percent had an A1C value of 8.0–9.0 percent.
  - 13.0 percent had an A1C value higher than 9.0 percent.
- 10.4 percent of adults aged 18–44 years had A1C levels of 10 percent or higher, compared to 9.4 percent of those aged 45–64 years and 2.6 percent of those aged 65 years or older.

High Blood Pressure

- 80.6 percent had a systolic blood pressure of 130 mmHg or higher or diastolic blood pressure of 80 mmHg or higher or were on prescription medication for their high blood pressure (HBP).
- 70.8 percent had a systolic blood pressure of 140 mmHg or higher or diastolic blood pressure of 90 mmHg or higher or were on prescription medication for their HBP.

High Cholesterol

- 39.5 percent had a non-HDL level of 130 mg/dL or higher. Specifically:
  - 19.9 percent had a non-HDL level of 130–159 mg/dL.
  - 11.5 percent had a non-HDL level of 160–189 mg/dL.
  - 8.0 percent had a non-HDL level of 190 mg/dL or higher.

PREVENTING DIABETES-RELATED COMPLICATIONS

Among U.S. adults aged 18 years or older with diagnosed diabetes, crude data for 2017–2020 indicated:

Usual Source for Diabetes Care

- 78.8 percent reported having at least one usual source of diabetes care, such as a doctor or other health-care professional.

Physical Activity

- 24.1 percent met the recommended goal of at least 150 minutes per week of leisure-time physical activity.

Weight Management

- 73.1 percent reported managing or losing weight to lower their risk for developing certain diseases.

Statin Treatment

- 57.8 percent of adults aged 40–75 years were on statin therapy.

A1C, Blood Pressure, Cholesterol, and Smoking (ABCs)

- 11.1 percent met all these criteria: A1C value <7.0 percent, blood pressure <130/80 mmHg, non-HDL cholesterol <130 mg/dL, and being a nonsmoker.
- 36.8 percent met all these criteria: A1C value <8.0 percent, blood pressure <140/90 mmHg, non-HDL cholesterol <160 mg/dL, and being a nonsmoker.

Vaccinations

Among U.S. adults aged 18 years or older with diagnosed diabetes, crude data for 2021 indicated:

- 65.9 percent (95% CI, 63.8–68.0) had received an influenza vaccination in the past year.
- 81.5 percent (95% CI, 79.4–83.4) had ever received a coronavirus 2019 (COVID-19) vaccination.

- 8.9 percent (95% CI, 7.6–10.4) had received one COVID-19 vaccination.
- 63.8 percent (95% CI, 61.5–66.1) had received two COVID-19 vaccinations.
- 8.7 percent (95% CI, 7.6–10.1) had received more than two COVID-19 vaccinations.
- 26.2 percent (95% CI, 24.2–28.3) had ever received a hepatitis B vaccination.
- 35.9 percent (95% CI, 32.2–39.8) of adults aged 18–59 years had ever received a hepatitis B vaccination.
- 50.7 percent (95% CI, 48.6–52.9) had ever received a pneumococcal vaccination.

The National Diabetes Statistics Report highlights the significant prevalence and incidence of diabetes and prediabetes in the United States. The data underscores the importance of addressing risk factors and preventing complications through effective management and public health interventions.[1]

[1] "National Diabetes Statistics Report," Centers for Disease Control and Prevention (CDC), May 15, 2024. Available online. URL: www.cdc.gov/diabetes/php/data-research/index.html. Accessed October 1, 2024.

Chapter 30 | Racial and Ethnic Disparities in Adult Obesity

COSTS OF OBESITY

Obesity is a problem for both children and adults in the United States. Nearly one in five young people aged 2–19 years have obesity. These children are at risk for type 2 diabetes, asthma, depression, and low self-esteem. The risk of adult obesity is also increased for individuals who had obesity as children.

Nearly 4 in 10 adults in the United States are obese. Adults with obesity often have multiple organ system complications from the condition and are more at risk for heart disease, stroke, type 2 diabetes, and 13 types of cancers. Obesity costs the United States health-care system approximately $147 billion a year. Adult obesity decreases productivity and increases the risk of workplace injuries. The cost of obesity-related absenteeism is between $3.4 billion and $6.4 billion each year. Obesity in young adults limits eligibility for many to serve in the military. About one in four young adults is too heavy to serve.

DISPARITIES

The Centers for Disease Control and Prevention (CDC) plays a key role in tracking data on the obesity burden and the racial and ethnic disparities within the obesity burden. The racial and ethnic maps for 2015–2017 show where obesity is more burdensome for particular populations. Overall, 31 states and the District of Columbia had an obesity prevalence of 35 percent or higher among non-Hispanic Black adults; 8 states (Arizona, Illinois, Kansas, Michigan, North

Dakota, Oklahoma, South Dakota, and Texas) had an obesity prevalence of 35 percent or higher among Hispanic adults; and only 1 state (West Virginia) had an obesity prevalence of 35 percent or higher among non-Hispanic white adults.

ENCOURAGING PHYSICAL ACTIVITY TO MANAGE AND PREVENT OBESITY

Physical activity has many other benefits beyond helping with weight management. Physical activity promotes health by reducing the risk of chronic diseases and other conditions that are often more common and more severe among racial and ethnic minority groups. Physical activity also fosters normal growth and development in children, improves mental health, and can make people feel better, function better, and sleep better. The *Physical Activity Guidelines for Americans, Second Edition* (https://health.gov/our-work/nutrition-physical-activity/physical-activity-guidelines/current-guidelines) outlines the amounts and types of physical activity needed to maintain or improve overall health and reduce the risk of chronic disease.

Despite the benefits of physical activity, too few Americans get the recommended amount. Only one in four adults and one in five high school students fully meet physical activity guidelines for aerobic and muscle-strengthening activities. These numbers are even lower among adults in some racial and ethnic minority populations.

One way communities can help residents be active is to create easy and safe options for physical activity. Since 1999, the CDC's Racial and Ethnic Approaches to Community Health (REACH) program (www.cdc.gov/reach/php/about/history.html) has demonstrated that through community participation, locally based and culturally tailored efforts can be effective. REACH communities address chronic diseases for specific racial and ethnic groups in urban, rural, and tribal communities with high disease burdens. They implement community planning and transportation plans that support safe and accessible physical activity by connecting sidewalks, paths, bike routes, and public transit with homes, early care and education settings, schools, and parks and recreation centers.

Racial and Ethnic Disparities in Adult Obesity

The CDC's State Physical Activity and Nutrition Program (SPAN; www.cdc.gov/span/php/about/index.html) and High Obesity Program (HOP; www.cdc.gov/hop/php/about/index.html) also focus on improving racial and ethnic health disparities and include strategies to increase physical activity. Through SPAN, the CDC funds statewide initiatives to implement evidence-based strategies at state and local levels to improve nutrition and physical activity. The CDC's HOP funds 15 land-grant universities to work with community extension services to increase access to healthier foods and safe and accessible places for physical activity in counties that have more than 40 percent of adults with obesity.[1]

[1] "Addressing Racial and Ethnic Health Disparities in Adult Obesity and Encouraging Physical Activity This National Minority Health Month," Centers for Disease Control and Prevention (CDC), April 24, 2019. Available online. URL: https://blogs.cdc.gov/healthequity/2019/04/24/addressing-racial-and-ethnic-health-disparities-in-adult-obesity-and-encouraging-physical-activity-this-national-minority-health-month. Accessed September 30, 2024.

Chapter 31 | Asthma Prevalence and Demographic Disparities

ASTHMA PREVALENCE AND DISPARITIES

Asthma is a chronic respiratory disease requiring ongoing medical management. Asthma has had a considerable economic effect and resulted in a substantial number of missed school days. In the United States, nearly 24.8 million people (7.7% of the population) had current asthma in 2018. Among children (individuals aged < 18 years), asthma was more prevalent among those in families with low incomes and among non-Hispanic Black children and those of Puerto Rican descent compared with non-Hispanic white children. Asthma has been associated with substantial morbidity and remains a focus of the U.S. Department of Health and Human Services (HHS) *Healthy People 2030* initiative.

GEOGRAPHIC DISPARITIES IN ASTHMA

Geographic disparities (e.g., regional, urban, and rural) in health outcomes have been documented, with higher numbers of excess deaths from chronic lower respiratory disease in rural areas than in urban areas. Socioeconomic and demographic factors (e.g., poverty, education status, age, race/ethnicity, sex, and insurance status) and health-care use might contribute to health outcome patterns observed in urban and rural areas. People living in rural areas typically have worse health outcomes and less access to health care than those in urban areas. Rural residents are more likely to live in areas with hospital closures, travel long distances to receive specialty or emergency care, and live in areas with shortages in the health-care workforce, subspecialty care, and preventative services; they are also less likely to have health insurance. Barriers to health-care access can result in unmet health-care needs and preventable hospitalizations. In contrast, suburban residents have been shown to have the best health outcomes.

SOCIAL DETERMINANTS OF HEALTH AND ASTHMA

Social determinants of health play a substantial role in health outcomes. Reducing racial and ethnic disparities in asthma risks and health care is of national strategic importance. Children, Black individuals, Hispanic individuals, people insured by Medicaid or the Children's Health Insurance Program (CHIP), and people living in the Northeast are more likely to visit an ED for asthma, which is a key indicator of poorly controlled asthma. Racial and ethnic health disparities among rural adults aged ≥ 18 years also have been reported. Limited health-care access and unmet health-care needs can result in serious life-threatening respiratory episodes and hinder timely access to ED care and survival.

TRENDS IN PREVALENCE OF CURRENT ASTHMA

During 2006–2018, overall and by metropolitan statistical area (MSA) category, current asthma prevalence among all ages and adults did not change significantly. However, among children, a decrease occurred in the overall trend, not considering MSA categories, in asthma prevalence (annual percent change [APC] = −1.6) and the trend in small MSAs (APC = −1.5).

PREVALENCE OF CURRENT ASTHMA BY DEMOGRAPHIC CHARACTERISTICS AND POVERTY LEVEL

Current asthma prevalence differed by demographic characteristics, regardless of MSA category. The difference in asthma prevalence between males and females varied by age group. Among children, boys had a higher prevalence (9.0%) than girls (7.1%), whereas among adults, women had a higher prevalence (10.0%) than men (5.7%). Current asthma prevalence was lowest among children aged 0–4 years (4.0%) and highest among those aged 12–17 years (10.5%). Among all ages, prevalence was higher among Black individuals (10.7%) and people of multiple races (13.1%) and lower among Asian (4.5%) and Hispanic individuals (6.5%) than among white individuals (8.0%). Among Hispanic individuals, Puerto Rican individuals had a higher prevalence of asthma (14.0%) than Mexican (5.4%) and other Hispanic individuals (6.3%).

Current asthma prevalence differed by poverty level.

PREVALENCE OF CURRENT ASTHMA BY GEOGRAPHIC LOCATION

Overall, the current asthma prevalence was higher in the Northeast (8.9%) than in the South (7.6%) and the West (7.7%); among adults, the current asthma prevalence was higher in the Northeast (8.8%) than in the South (7.4%). Among children, the prevalence was higher in the Northeast (9.1%) than in the West (6.9%).

The prevalence of current asthma overall and among adults was higher in small MSAs (all ages: 8.4%; adults: 8.3%) than in large MSAs (all ages: 7.7%; adults: 7.7%). In the small MSA areas, asthma prevalence was higher in the Northeast (10.2%) than in the South (7.8%). Among urban-rural classification categories, the prevalence was higher in the medium metropolitan areas (8.5%) and small metropolitan areas (8.4%) than in large central metropolitan areas (7.3%).

The prevalence of people with current asthma varied by state. The prevalence differed by MSA category in California, Colorado, Mississippi, Oklahoma, and Tennessee but not by the same patterns in each state. In California, asthma prevalence was higher in non-MSAs (11.2%) than in large MSAs (6.4%), whereas in Colorado, the prevalence was higher in small MSAs (10.9%) than in non-MSAs (6.6%). In Mississippi, the prevalence was higher in small MSAs (9.3%) than in large MSAs (3.2%) and non-MSAs (5.0%), and in Oklahoma, the prevalence was higher in large MSAs (10.6%) than in small MSAs (5.3%). In Tennessee, the prevalence was higher in small MSAs (8.7%) and in non-MSAs (8.3%) than in large MSAs (4.5%).

Addressing these disparities through targeted public health initiatives and improving access to health-care services is essential for reducing the burden of asthma and improving health outcomes for affected individuals.[1]

[1] "Asthma Surveillance — United States, 2006–2018," Centers for Disease Control and Prevention (CDC), September 16, 2021. Available online. URL: www.cdc.gov/mmwr/volumes/70/ss/ss7005a1.htm?s_cid=ss7005a1_w. Accessed October 1, 2024.

Chapter 32 | COPD Prevalence and Disparities across Sociodemographic Groups

Chronic obstructive pulmonary disease (COPD) is a group of progressive lung diseases, including emphysema and chronic bronchitis. COPD accounts for most deaths from chronic lower respiratory diseases, the sixth leading cause of death in the United States in 2021. Elevated prevalence of COPD has been reported in the following groups: women, older adults (aged ≥ 65 years), residents in rural areas, adults with a lower education level, and those who have ever smoked. During 1999–2011, estimates from the National Health Interview Survey (NHIS) indicated that the prevalence of self-reported physician-diagnosed COPD significantly declined among U.S. adults (aged ≥ 25 years) overall and among adults aged 25–44 years. Trends and differences in COPD prevalence during the previous decade have not been reported overall and by subgroups.

DIFFERENCES BY SOCIODEMOGRAPHIC CHARACTERISTICS

An estimated 6.4 percent of U.S. adults (population estimate = 14.3 million) in 2011 and 6.5 percent (14.2 million) in 2021 had COPD. In 2011 and 2021, age-standardized COPD prevalence was higher among women than among men, higher among non-Hispanic American Indian or Alaska Native and non-Hispanic other individuals than among non-Hispanic white individuals, higher among people who were unemployed, retired, homemakers or students, and unable to work than among those who were employed, and higher among adults who were current or former smokers than among never-smokers. Prevalence was lower among non-Hispanic Asian, Native Hawaiian, Pacific-Islander, or Hispanic individuals than among non-Hispanic white individuals.

TRENDS OVER TIME

The age-standardized prevalence of COPD from 2011 to 2021 remained stable overall (6.1% in 2011 to 6.0% in 2021) and for most subgroups. COPD prevalence increased significantly from 2011 to 2018 and remained stable from 2018 to 2021 among adults aged 45–64 and those living in noncore areas. Age-standardized COPD prevalence in 2011 ranged from 3.9 percent in Minnesota to 9.5 percent in Kentucky, and in 2021, from 3 percent in Hawaii to 11.8 percent in West Virginia.

An estimated 14.2 million (6.5%) U.S. adults had physician-diagnosed COPD in 2021. These results are consistent with overall COPD mortality rates, which remained unchanged during 1999–2019. The prevalence of COPD among adults aged < 45 years declined from 2011 to 2021, consistent with the trend during 1999–2011. One reason might be the more pronounced decline in the prevalence of current smoking among adults aged 18–44 years (36.4% relative decline) than among those aged 45–64 years (22.6%) and those aged ≥ 65 years (2.1%) from 2005 to 2015; cigarette smoking is the dominant cause of COPD among U.S. adults. Explanations for the higher prevalence of COPD among those living in micropolitan and noncore counties might include the persistently high prevalence of smoking among adults in rural areas, the lower rates of people quitting smoking, and the increasing proportion of older adults living in rural areas. The variation in the prevalence of COPD by states is likely related to factors including differences in smoking rates, occupations or industries with higher risk for COPD, and access to health care for screening and detection of COPD.

Approximately, 25 percent of adults with COPD (3.8 million) reported having never smoked, similar to 1988–1994. In addition to cigarette smoking, secondhand smoke and occupational and environmental exposures are also risk factors for developing COPD among nonsmokers.

IMPLICATIONS FOR PUBLIC HEALTH PRACTICE

The COPD National Action Plan provides a comprehensive framework for developing and implementing COPD prevention, treatment, and management strategies. Patient and population-based initiatives focusing on COPD prevention (e.g., smoking cessation, smoke-free policies, and workplace interventions), early diagnosis, treatment (e.g., medication and oxygen therapy), and management (e.g., access to pulmonary rehabilitation and caregiving, efforts to prevent exacerbations) might reduce COPD prevalence, slow the progression of the disease, and lessen symptoms. Strategies can be tailored to address the prevention of COPD-related risk factors and the needs of adults disproportionately affected by COPD, including older people aged ≥ 75 years, those who have ever smoked, and residents of rural areas. For example, residents of rural areas have less access to pulmonologists. Implementation of COPD programs designed for rural communities can address the challenges that people from these areas face, including higher prevalence of tobacco use, cultural barriers, poverty, and lack of specialists or transportation.[1]

[1] "Trends in the Prevalence of Chronic Obstructive Pulmonary Disease among Adults Aged ≥18 Years — United States, 2011–2021," Centers for Disease Control and Prevention (CDC), November 16, 2023. Available online. URL: www.cdc.gov/mmwr/volumes/72/wr/mm7246a1.htm. Accessed October 1, 2024.

Chapter 33 | **Cancer and Demographic Variations**

Chapter Contents

Section 33.1 | Cancer Disparities across Populations and Contributing Factors

CANCER DISPARITIES

Cancer is a disease in which some of the body's cells grow uncontrollably and spread to other parts of the body.

Cancer affects all population groups in the United States, but due to social, environmental, and economic disadvantages, certain groups bear a disproportionate burden of cancer compared with other groups.

Cancer disparities (sometimes referred to as "cancer health disparities") are differences in cancer measures such as:

- incidence (new cases)
- prevalence (all existing cases)
- mortality (deaths)
- survival (how long people survive after diagnosis)
- morbidity (cancer-related health complications)
- survivorship (including quality of life after cancer treatment)
- the financial burden of cancer or related health conditions
- screening rates
- stage at diagnosis

Cancer disparities can also be seen when outcomes are improving overall but the improvements are not seen in some groups relative to other groups.

Population groups that may experience cancer disparities include groups defined by race, ethnicity, disability, gender identity, geographic location, income, education, age, sexual orientation, national origin, and other characteristics.

EXAMPLES OF CANCER DISPARITIES

Although cancer incidence and mortality overall are declining in all population groups in the United States, some groups continue to be at increased risk of developing or dying from certain cancers.

Statistics from the National Cancer Institute's (NCI) Surveillance, Epidemiology, and End Results (SEER) Program include information specific to racial and ethnic groups as well as populations defined by age, gender, and geography. Some key cancer incidence and mortality disparities in the United States are as follows:

- Black/African-American individuals have higher death rates than all other racial/ethnic groups for many, although not all, cancer types.
- Black/African-American women are more likely than white women to die from breast cancer, despite having slightly lower incidence rates.
- People living in rural Appalachia have much higher incidence rates of colorectal, lung, and cervical cancers compared to those living in urban areas within the region.
- Black/African-American men are more than twice as likely as white men to die from prostate cancer and continue to have the highest prostate cancer mortality rates among all U.S. racial/ethnic groups, even though deaths from prostate cancer have decreased substantially among all men in recent decades.
- Individuals with higher education levels are less likely to die prematurely (before the age of 65) from colorectal cancer than those with less education, regardless of race or ethnicity.
- Hispanic/Latino, Black/African-American, and American Indian/Alaska Native women have higher incidence rates of cervical cancer than women of other racial/ethnic groups, with Black/African-American women experiencing the highest death rates from the disease.
- American Indians/Alaska Natives have higher death rates from kidney cancer than any other racial/ethnic group.
- Lesbian, gay, and bisexual (LGB) youths have higher rates of smoking and alcohol consumption, which increase cancer risk, compared to heterosexual youths.

- American Indians/Alaska Natives also have the highest incidence and mortality rates of liver and intrahepatic bile duct cancer, followed by Hispanics/Latinos and Asians/Pacific Islanders.

CONTRIBUTING FACTORS

Cancer disparities reflect the interplay among many factors, including social determinants of health, behavior, biology, and genetics—all of which can have profound effects on health, including cancer risk and outcomes.

Certain groups in the United States experience cancer disparities because they are more likely to encounter obstacles in getting health care.

For example, people with low incomes, low health literacy, long travel distances to screening or treatment sites, or who lack health insurance, transportation to a medical facility, or paid medical leave are less likely to have recommended cancer screening tests and to be treated according to guidelines than those who do not encounter these obstacles.

People who do not have reliable access to health care are also more likely to be diagnosed with late-stage cancer, which might have been treated more effectively if it had been diagnosed at an earlier stage.

Some groups are disproportionately affected by cancer due to environmental conditions. People who live in communities that lack clean water or air may be exposed to cancer-causing substances.

The built environment can also influence behaviors that raise one's risk of cancer. For example, people who live in neighborhoods that lack affordable healthy foods or safe areas for exercise are more likely to have poor diets, be physically inactive, and be obese, all of which are risk factors for cancer.

Even people of higher socioeconomic status and those with health insurance may experience cancer disparities. The disparities these individuals experience may reflect the health effects of institutional racism and the chronic stress it causes, conscious or unconscious bias from health providers, mistrust of the health-care system, or fatalistic attitudes about cancer.

In some cases, inherited factors or tumor biological factors may, either directly or by interacting with factors such as diet, chronic stress, or tobacco exposure, lead to cancer disparities.

For example, some evidence suggests that there are differences in the genetics, tumor biology, and immune environment of several cancers that arise in Black/African Americans compared with those that arise in people of other racial/ethnic groups. These differences may contribute to disparities in incidence, cancer growth rate, and response to treatment of these cancers.

Cancer disparities may also be exacerbated by the lack of diversity in clinical research participation. Because of this lack of diversity, research results may not be applicable to all populations.

Because many different factors can influence cancer disparities, addressing them is not simple or straightforward. Reducing or eliminating some cancer disparities in the pursuit of health equity will require policy changes to overcome systemic social, racial, and institutional inequalities.[1]

Section 33.2 | Disparities in Common Cancer Incidence across Demographic Groups

CANCER INCIDENCE

Cancer incidence is typically measured as the number of new cases each year for every 100,000 people (for sex-specific cancers, people of the same sex serve as the denominator) and age-adjusted to a standard population to allow comparisons over time.

PROJECTED CANCER CASES FOR 2024

In 2024, nearly half of all new cancer cases are expected to be cancers of the prostate, breast, lung, and colon and rectum. According to American Cancer Society (www.cancer.org) projections, about

[1] "Cancer Disparities," National Cancer Institute (NCI), March 21, 2024. Available online. URL: www.cancer.gov/about-cancer/understanding/disparities. Accessed October 3, 2024.

2,001,140 new cases of cancer are expected to be diagnosed in 2024, including:

- 299,010 cases of prostate cancer
- 313,510 cases of breast cancer
- 234,580 cases of lung and bronchus cancer
- 152,810 cases of colorectal cancer

TRENDS AND MOST RECENT ESTIMATES

Confidence interval indicates the range of values expected for the true estimate to fall between if the study were to be redone many times. If a study has 95 percent confidence interval calculated, then this means that if the study was repeated multiple times with samples from the whole population and the confidence intervals were calculated for each of those repeated studies, then the true value would lie within the calculated confidence intervals 95 percent of the time.

All Cancer Sites Combined—By Sex

Table 33.1 provides the most recent estimates of delay-adjusted cancer incidence rates per 100,000 population, categorized by sex.

Table 33.1. Rates of New Cases of All Cancer, Delay-Adjusted Cancer Incidence by Sex, 1975–2021

	Most Recent Estimates (2021)	
Sex	**Rate per 100,000**	**95% Confidence Interval**
Both sexes	461.4	459.0–463.9
Male	492.8	489.2–496.4
Female	443.2	439.9–446.5

Source: NCI, 2021.

All Cancer Sites Combined—By Race/Ethnicity

Table 33.2 provides the most recent estimates of delay-adjusted cancer incidence rates per 100,000 population, categorized by race and ethnicity.

Table 33.2. Rates of New Cases of All Cancer, Delay-Adjusted Cancer Incidence by Race/Ethnicity, 2000–2021

	Most Recent Estimates (2021)	
Race/Ethnicity	**Rate per 100,000**	**95% Confidence Interval**
All races	458.3	457.3–459.3
Non-Hispanic white	467.5	466.3–468.6
Non-Hispanic Black	461.7	458.6–464.7
Hispanic	372.8	370.5–375.0
Non-Hispanic Asian/Pacific Islander	329.7	326.8–332.5
Non-Hispanic American Indian/Alaska Native	477.9	459.1–497.2

Source: NCI, 2021.

Comparison of Top Cancer Sites

Table 33.3 provides the most recent estimates of delay-adjusted cancer incidence rates per 100,000 population for the most common cancers.

Table 33.3. Rates of New Cases of the Most Common Cancers, Delay-Adjusted Cancer Incidence, 1975–2021

	Most Recent Estimates (2021)	
Common Cancer	**Rate per 100,000**	**95% Confidence Interval**
Colon and Rectum	35.8	35.2–36.5
Lung and Bronchus	43.7	43.0–44.4
Female breast	144.6	142.7–146.5
Prostate	131.4	129.6–133.3

Source: NCI, 2021.

Colon and Rectum Cancer—By Sex

Table 33.4 provides the most recent estimates of delay-adjusted cancer incidence rates per 100,000 population for colon and rectum cancer, categorized by sex.

Table 33.4. Rates of New Cases of Colon and Rectum Cancer, Delay-Adjusted Cancer Incidence by Sex, 1975–2021

	Most Recent Estimates (2021)	
Sex	**Rate per 100,000**	**95% Confidence Interval**
Both sexes	35.8	35.2–36.5
Male	39.9	38.9–41.0
Female	32.2	31.3–33.1

Source: NCI, 2021.

Colon and Rectum Cancer—By Race/Ethnicity

Table 33.5 provides the most recent 2021 estimates of delay-adjusted cancer incidence rates per 100,000 population for colon and rectum cancer, categorized by race and ethnicity.

Table 33.5. Rates of New Cases of Colon and Rectum Cancer, Delay-Adjusted Cancer Incidence by Race/Ethnicity, 2000–2021

	Most Recent Estimates (2021)	
Race/Ethnicity	**Rate per 100,000**	**95% Confidence Interval**
All races	37.5	37.2–37.8
Non-Hispanic white	37.1	36.8–37.4
Non-Hispanic Black	41.9	41.0–42.8
Hispanic	35.3	34.6–36.0
Non-Hispanic Asian/ Pacific Islander	31.3	30.4–32.2
Non-Hispanic American Indian/ Alaska Native	58.6	52.1–65.6

Source: NCI, 2021.

Lung and Bronchus Cancer—By Sex

Table 33.6 provides the most recent estimates of delay-adjusted cancer incidence rates per 100,000 population for lung and bronchus cancer, categorized by sex.

Table 33.6. Rates of New Cases of Lung and Bronchus Cancer, Delay-Adjusted Cancer Incidence by Sex, 1975–2021

	Most Recent Estimates (2021)	
Sex	**Rate per 100,000**	**95% Confidence Interval**
Both sexes	43.7	43.0–44.4
Male	46.7	45.6–47.8
Female	41.6	40.6–42.6

Source: NCI, 2021.

Lung and Bronchus Cancer—By Race/Ethnicity

Table 33.7 provides the most recent estimates of delay-adjusted cancer incidence rates per 100,000 population for lung and bronchus cancer, categorized by race and ethnicity.

Table 33.7. Rates of New Cases of Lung and Bronchus Cancer, Delay-Adjusted Cancer Incidence by Race/Ethnicity, 2000–2021

	Most Recent Estimates (2021)	
Race/Ethnicity	**Rate per 100,000**	**95% Confidence Interval**
All races	46.9	46.6–47.3
Non-Hispanic white	48.1	47.8–48.5
Non-Hispanic Black	48.6	47.6–49.6
Hispanic	25.5	24.9–26.2
Non-Hispanic Asian/ Pacific Islander	33.5	32.6–34.4
Non-Hispanic American Indian/Alaska Native	57.5	51.1–64.3

Source: NCI, 2021.

Female Breast Cancer—By Race/Ethnicity

Table 33.8 provides the most recent estimates of delay-adjusted cancer incidence rates per 100,000 population for female breast cancer, categorized by race and ethnicity.

Table 33.8. Rates of New Cases of Female Breast Cancer, Delay-Adjusted Cancer Incidence by Race/Ethnicity, 2000–2021

	Most Recent Estimates (2021)	
Race/Ethnicity	**Rate per 100,000**	**95% Confidence Interval**
All races	137.4	136.6–138.2
Non-Hispanic white	138.7	137.8–139.6
Non-Hispanic Black	131.1	128.9–133.3
Hispanic	111.1	109.5–112.7
Non-Hispanic Asian/ Pacific Islander	125.5	123.1–127.9
Non-Hispanic American Indian/Alaska Native	131.0	117.8–145.2

Source: NCI, 2021.

Prostate Cancer—By Race/Ethnicity

Table 33.9 provides the most recent estimates of delay-adjusted cancer incidence rates per 100,000 population for prostate cancer, categorized by race and ethnicity.[1]

Table 33.9. Rates of New Cases of Prostate Cancer, Delay-Adjusted Cancer Incidence by Race/Ethnicity, 2000–2021

	Most Recent Estimates (2021)	
Race/Ethnicity	**Rate per 100,000**	**95% Confidence Interval**
All races	128.0	127.2–128.7
Non-Hispanic white	121.1	120.3–122.0

[1] "Incidence—Cancer Trends Progress Report," National Cancer Institute (NCI), August 2024. Available online. URL: https://progressreport.cancer.gov/diagnosis/incidence. Accessed October 3, 2024.

Table 33.9. Continued

Race/Ethnicity	Most Recent Estimates (2021)	
	Rate per 100,000	**95% Confidence Interval**
Non-Hispanic Black	209.8	206.6–213.0
Hispanic	96.3	94.5–98.1
Non-Hispanic Asian/ Pacific Islander	71.3	69.3–73.3
Non-Hispanic American Indian/Alaska Native	101.5	88.5–115.8

Source: NCI, 2021.

Section 33.3 | Emerging Biomarkers for Cancer Risk and Early Detection

THE SEARCH FOR CANCER BIOMARKERS

For many years, scientists have sought to identify biological markers, or biomarkers, that accurately indicate an increased risk of cancer or the presence of early stage disease. The identification of increased risk may provide an opportunity for medical intervention to reduce risk or heightened surveillance and early intervention as needed. Earlier cancer detection may permit earlier, more effective treatment and increase the chances of long-term survival. Biomarkers may also allow differentiation between cancers, precursor lesions that need to be treated, and precursor lesions that would never cause symptoms or threaten life and, therefore, do not need to be treated.

Biomarkers include genetic mutations, other changes in DNA (deoxyribonucleic acid), and abnormalities in proteins or other biological molecules that indicate the presence of an anomaly. They may be detected in blood, stool, other body fluids, or tissue. It is known that inherited mutations in certain genes, such as *BRCA1* and *BRCA2*, which can be detected in blood samples, confer high risks of breast and ovarian cancers, but inherited mutations account for only a small percentage of all cancers that occur.

Although numerous biomarkers of cancer risk or malignant disease have been reported in the scientific literature in recent decades, very few have been validated or shown to be clinically useful. This fact led the Institute of Medicine and other organizations to develop recommendations and frameworks for cancer biomarker development.

These recommendations are crucial and timely because our ever-increasing understanding of the mechanisms of cancer, greatly facilitated by advanced genomic, proteomic, and other molecular technologies, is amplifying opportunities for cancer biomarker discovery and development. Moreover, biomarkers that reflect mechanisms related to cancer development or growth may suggest targeted chemoprevention to inhibit these mechanisms, which could form the basis of precision prevention and treatment.

CIRCULATING TUMOR DNA AS A NEW BIOMARKER

Many malignant tumors shed entire cells, fragments of cells, and intracellular molecules into their immediate environment early in the disease process. Often, these substances are detectable in the blood, other body fluids, or feces, providing the potential for easier, less invasive screening methods for early cancer detection.

One type of biomarker that has been the focus of much interest lately is tumor cell DNA circulating in the blood, also known as "circulating tumor DNA" (ctDNA). This DNA is marked by key mutations or other abnormalities found in the DNA of intact tumor cells.

In an international study involving 640 participants reported in 2014, researchers, including members of the National Cancer Institute's (NCI) Early Detection Research Network, used state-of-the-art molecular techniques to detect ctDNA in patients with various types of early- or late-stage cancer. Among patients with early stage cancer, detectable ctDNA was found in 47 percent of those with stage I disease and 55 percent of those with stage II disease. Among patients with late-stage cancer, ctDNA was detected in 69 percent of the individuals with stage III disease and 82 percent of the individuals with stage IV disease.

Although these findings are promising, a number of technical challenges, including increasing the sensitivity of ctDNA detection, must be overcome before ctDNA assays can be applied clinically. Another challenge is that, theoretically, ctDNA may be released by a tumor before the tumor can be detected definitively with current imaging technologies, raising questions about how patients with detectable ctDNA but no tumor detectable by imaging would be managed medically.

EXOSOMES AS EMERGING BIOMARKERS

Exosomes are another type of biomarker currently under investigation. They are extracellular, nano-sized vesicles (tiny membrane-enclosed cell fragments) that contain proteins, DNA, and RNA. All cells, including cancer cells, release exosomes. These tiny vesicles can enter the bloodstream and travel throughout the body. Over the past decade, researchers have been exploring the use of exosomes as potential biomarkers for various diseases, including cancer.

In 2015, NCI-supported researchers reported that a protein called "glypican 1" (GPC1), which is abundantly expressed on the surface of breast and pancreatic cancer cells, is also found on the surface of most exosomes derived from these cells. The presence of GPC1 on exosomes derived from normal breast and pancreatic cells is rare. The researchers then developed a method for detecting exosomes in blood and examined the blood of 190 patients with pancreatic cancer, 32 patients with breast cancer, and 100 healthy donors. In comparison with the healthy donors, all patients with pancreatic cancer and 75 percent of patients with breast cancer had higher levels of GPC1-containing exosomes in their blood.

Additional preliminary experiments suggest that GPC1 might be a marker for early pancreatic disease. Blood levels of GPC1-containing exosomes were consistently higher among five patients with pancreatic cancer precursor lesions than among healthy donors or 26 patients with benign pancreatic disease, such as chronic pancreatitis. The researchers validated their findings in an independent group of patients that included six with chronic pancreatitis, 56 with pancreatic cancer, and 20 healthy donors.

If these preliminary findings are confirmed, the results raise the possibility that a noninvasive screening test to detect pancreatic cancer early may be possible, opening the door to potentially curative surgery or the development of other new therapeutic interventions for more patients diagnosed with this frequently fatal disease.

THE FUTURE OF BIOMARKER RESEARCH AND CANCER PREVENTION

The research and applications described above, both realized and potential, represent only a small fraction of the NCI's efforts to advance cancer prevention and early detection. This work and these intriguing possibilities have been bolstered by our increasing knowledge and understanding of cancer and the advanced technologies that are ushering in a new era of precision medicine.[1]

[1] "Improved Strategies for Cancer Prevention and Early Detection," National Cancer Institute (NCI), September 11, 2015. Available online. URL: www.cancer.gov/research/progress/discovery/strategies-prevention-early-detection#biomarkers. Accessed October 3, 2024.

Chapter 34 | Chronic Liver Disease

Chapter Contents

Section 34.1 | Chronic Liver Disease and African Americans

HOW DOES CHRONIC LIVER DISEASE AFFECT AFRICAN-AMERICAN POPULATIONS?

According to the Centers for Disease Control and Prevention (CDC), chronic liver disease includes health problems that affect the liver over time. The liver is the body's largest internal organ. It lies under the ribs on the right side of the abdomen. The liver performs many important functions, including removing waste from the body, such as toxins and medicines, making bile to help digest food, storing sugar that the body uses for energy, and producing new proteins. Liver disease affects the way the liver functions.

Chronic liver disease is a significant problem in the African-American population. While the cause of chronic liver disease is not always known, some cases can be initiated by conditions such as chronic alcoholism and exposure to hepatitis B and C viruses.

- In 2020, chronic liver disease was the ninth leading cause of death for non-Hispanic Black individuals aged 45–64 years old.
- African-American/Black men are 60 percent more likely to have liver and intrahepatic bile duct (IBD) cancer and to die from this disease compared to non-Hispanic white men.
- African-American/Black women are 30 percent more likely to die from liver and IBD cancer than non-Hispanic white women.

CANCER RATES (2015–2019)

Table 34.1 provides cancer incidence rates per 100,000 for non-Hispanic Black and non-Hispanic white men.

Table 34.1. Cancer Incidence Rates per 100,000—Men

Cancer	Non-Hispanic Black Men	Non-Hispanic White Men	Non-Hispanic Black/ Non-Hispanic White Ratio
All sites	535.1	514.8	1.0
Liver and IBD	18.1	11.3	1.6

Source: NCI, 2022.

Table 34.2 provides cancer incidence rates per 100,000 for non-Hispanic Black and non-Hispanic white women.

Table 34.2. Cancer Incidence Rates per 100,000—Women

Cancer	Non-Hispanic Black Women	Non-Hispanic White Women	Non-Hispanic Black/ Non-Hispanic White Ratio
All sites	408.7	450.8	0.9
Liver and IBD	5.5	4.1	1.3

Source: NCI, 2022.

DIAGNOSED

Table 34.3 provides the age-adjusted percentage of adults aged 18 and over who have been diagnosed with chronic liver disease, comparing non-Hispanic Black and non-Hispanic white populations.

Table 34.3. Age-Adjusted Percentage of Adults Aged 18 and Over Who Have Been Told by a Doctor That They Have Chronic Liver Disease, 2018

Non-Hispanic Black	Non-Hispanic White	Non-Hispanic Black/ Non-Hispanic White Ratio
1.1	1.6	0.7

Source: CDC, 2022.

DEATH RATES (2016–2020)

Table 34.4 provides cancer death rates per 100,000 for non-Hispanic Black and non-Hispanic white men.

Table 34.4. Cancer Death Rates per 100,000—Men

Cancer	Non-Hispanic Black Men	Non-Hispanic White Men	Non-Hispanic Black/ Non-Hispanic White Ratio
All sites	216.0	182.5	1.2
Liver and IBD	12.9	8.4	1.5

Source: NCI, 2022.

Table 34.5 provides cancer death rates per 100,000 for non-Hispanic Black and non-Hispanic white women.

Table 34.5. Cancer Death Rates per 100,000—Women

Cancer	Non-Hispanic Black Women	Non-Hispanic White Women	Non-Hispanic Black/ Non-Hispanic White Ratio
All sites	149.2	133.0	1.1
Liver and IBD	4.8	3.6	1.3

Source: NCI, 2022.

Table 34.6 provides the age-adjusted death rates for chronic liver disease and cirrhosis per 100,000 population, comparing non-Hispanic Black and non-Hispanic white women.[1]

Table 34.6. Age-Adjusted Chronic Liver Disease and Cirrhosis Death Rates per 100,000 (2019)

Sex	Non-Hispanic Black	Non-Hispanic White	Non-Hispanic Black/ Non-Hispanic White Ratio
Men	10.4	15.4	0.7

[1] Office of Minority Health (OMH), "Chronic Liver Disease and African Americans," U.S. Department of Health and Human Services (HHS), 2022. Available online. URL: https://minorityhealth.hhs.gov/chronic-liver-disease-and-african-americans. Accessed October 1, 2024.

Table 34.6. Continued

Sex	Non-Hispanic Black	Non-Hispanic White	Non-Hispanic Black/ Non-Hispanic White Ratio
Women	5.5	8.7	0.6
Total	7.7	11.9	0.6

Source: CDC, 2022.

Section 34.2 | Chronic Liver Disease and American Indians/Alaska Natives

HOW DOES CHRONIC LIVER DISEASE AFFECT AMERICAN INDIANS/ALASKA NATIVES?

According to the Centers for Disease Control and Prevention (CDC), chronic liver disease includes health problems that affect the liver over time. The liver is the body's largest internal organ. It lies under the ribs on the right side of the abdomen. The liver performs many important functions, including removing waste from the body, such as toxins and medicines, making bile to help digest food, storing sugar that the body uses for energy, and producing new proteins. Liver disease affects the way the liver functions.

Among American Indians/Alaska Natives, chronic liver disease is a leading cause of death. While the cause is not always known, some cases can be initiated by conditions such as chronic alcoholism, obesity, and exposure to hepatitis B and C viruses.

- In 2019, chronic liver disease was the fourth leading cause of death for all American Indians/Alaska Natives and the second leading cause of death for American Indian/Alaska Native men aged 35–44 years.
- In 2018, American Indians/Alaska Natives were 1.6 times more likely to be diagnosed with chronic liver disease compared to non-Hispanic whites.
- The overall death rate for American Indians/Alaska Natives is almost four times higher than the non-Hispanic white population.

- American Indian/Alaska Native women are 2.2 times as likely to be diagnosed with chronic liver disease and 4.8 times more likely to die from chronic liver disease compared to non-Hispanic white women.

CANCER RATES (2014–2018)

Table 34.7 provides cancer incidence rates per 100,000 for non-Hispanic Black men, non-Hispanic white men, and American Indian/Alaska Native men.

Table 34.7. Cancer Incidence Rates per 100,000—Men

Cancer	Non-Hispanic Black Men	Non-Hispanic White Men	American Indian/Alaska Native/ Non-Hispanic White Ratio
All sites	326.7	520.4	0.7
Liver and IBD	21.7	11.3	1.9

Source: NCI, 2021.

Table 34.8 provides cancer incidence rates per 100,000 for non-Hispanic Black women, non-Hispanic white women, and American Indian/Alaska Native women.

Table 34.8. Cancer Incidence Rates per 100,000—Women

Cancer	Non-Hispanic Black Women	Non-Hispanic White Women	American Indian/Alaska Native/ Non-Hispanic White Ratio
All sites	311.1	460.2	0.7
Liver and IBD	8.6	4.0	2.2

Source: NCI, 2021.

DIAGNOSED

Table 34.9 provides the age-adjusted percentage of adults aged 18 and over who have been diagnosed with chronic liver disease, comparing American Indian/Alaska Native and non-Hispanic white populations.

Table 34.9. Age-Adjusted Percentage of Adults Aged 18 and Over Who Have Been Told by a Doctor That They Have Chronic Liver Disease, 2018

American Indian/ Alaska Native	Non-Hispanic White	American Indian/ Alaska Native/ Non-Hispanic White Ratio
2.5	1.6	1.6

Source: CDC, 2020.

DEATH RATES (2014–2018)

Table 34.10 provides cancer death rates per 100,000 for American Indian/Alaska Native men and non-Hispanic white men.

Table 34.10. Cancer Death Rates per 100,000—Men

Cancer	American Indian/ Alaska Native Men	Non-Hispanic White Men	American Indian/ Alaska Native/ Non-Hispanic White Ratio
All sites	169.3	190.2	0.9
Liver and IBD	14.8	8.4	1.8

Source: NCI, 2021.

Table 34.11 provides cancer death rates per 100,000 for American Indian/Alaska Native women and non-Hispanic white women.

Table 34.11. Cancer Death Rates per 100,000—Women

Cancer	American Indian/ Alaska Native Women	Non-Hispanic White Women	American Indian/ Alaska Native/ Non-Hispanic White Ratio
All sites	120.1	137.8	0.9
Liver and IBD	7.0	3.6	1.9

Source: NCI, 2021.

Table 34.12 provides age-adjusted death rates per 100,000 for chronic liver disease and cirrhosis, comparing non-Hispanic American Indian/Alaska Native and non-Hispanic white populations.[1]

Table 34.12. Age-Adjusted Chronic Liver Disease and Cirrhosis Death Rates per 100,000 (2018)

Sex	Non-Hispanic American Indian/Alaska Native	Non-Hispanic White	Non-Hispanic American Indian/Alaska Native/ Non-Hispanic White Ratio
Men	506	14.9	3.4
Women	40.2	8.3	4.8
Total	45.2	11.5	3.9

Source: CDC, 2021.

Section 34.3 | **Chronic Liver Disease and Asian Americans**

HOW DOES CHRONIC LIVER DISEASE AFFECT ASIAN AMERICANS?

According to the Centers for Disease Control and Prevention (CDC), chronic liver disease includes health problems that affect the liver over time. The liver is the body's largest internal organ. It lies under the ribs on the right side of the abdomen. The liver performs many important functions, including removing waste from the body, such as toxins and medicines, making bile to help digest food, storing sugar that the body uses for energy, and producing new proteins. Liver disease affects the way the liver functions.

Among Asian Americans, chronic liver disease is a leading cause of death. While the exact cause is not always known, some cases

[1] Office of Minority Health (OMH), "Chronic Liver Disease and American Indians/Alaska Natives," U.S. Department of Health and Human Services (HHS), 2021. Available online. URL: https://minorityhealth.hhs.gov/chronic-liver-disease-and-american-indiansalaska-natives. Accessed October 1, 2024.

can be initiated by conditions such as chronic alcoholism, obesity, and exposure to hepatitis B and C viruses.

- In 2019, chronic liver disease was the sixth leading cause of death for Asian/Pacific Islanders aged 25–44 years.
- Asian-American men have higher incidence rates of liver cancer compared to Hispanic, non-Hispanic white, or Asian/Pacific-Islander men.
- Asian male subgroups exhibit higher mortality rates for liver cancer, specifically:
  - 54.3 for Vietnamese
  - 33.9 for Koreans
  - 23.3 for Chinese
  - 16.8 for Filipino
  - 9.3 for Japanese
- Asian-American men are 60 percent more likely to die from liver and intrahepatic bile duct (IBD) cancer compared to non-Hispanic white men.
- The incidence rate for liver and IBD cancer is 1.8 times higher for Asian-American women compared to non-Hispanic white women.

CANCER RATES (2014–2018)

Table 34.13 provides cancer incidence rates per 100,000 for Asian/Pacific-Islander men and non-Hispanic white men.

Table 34.13. Cancer Incidence Rates per 100,000—Men

Cancer	Asian/Pacific-Islander Men	Non-Hispanic White Men	Asian/Pacific Islander/Non-Hispanic White Ratio
All sites	309.1	520.4	0.6
Liver and IBD	19.4	11.3	1.7

Source: NCI, 2021.

Table 34.14 provides cancer incidence rates per 100,000 for Asian/Pacific-Islander women and non-Hispanic white women.

Table 34.14. Cancer Incidence Rates per 100,000—Women

Cancer	Asian/Pacific-Islander Women	Non-Hispanic White Women	Asian/Pacific-Islander/ Non-Hispanic White Ratio
All sites	311.5	460.2	0.7
Liver and IBD	7.1	4.0	1.9

Source: NCI, 2021.

DIAGNOSED

Table 34.15 provides the age-adjusted percentage of adults aged 18 and over who have been diagnosed with chronic liver disease, comparing Asian/Pacific-Islander and non-Hispanic white populations.

Table 34.15. Age-Adjusted Percentage of Adults Aged 18 and Over Who Have Been Told by a Doctor That They Have Chronic Liver Disease, 2018

Asian/Pacific Islander	Non-Hispanic White	Asian/Pacific-Islander/ Non-Hispanic White Ratio
1.1	1.6	0.7

Source: CDC, 2020.

DEATH RATES (2014–2018)

Table 34.16 provides cancer death rates per 100,000 for Asian/ Pacific-Islander men and non-Hispanic white men.

Table 34.16. Cancer Death Rates per 100,000—Men

Cancer	Asian/Pacific-Islander Men	Non-Hispanic White Men	Asian/Pacific-Islander/ Non-Hispanic White Ratio
All sites	114.6	190.2	0.6
Liver and IBD	13.1	8.4	1.6

Source: NCI, 2021.

Table 34.17 provides cancer death rates per 100,000 for Asian/ Pacific-Islander women and non-Hispanic white women.

Table 34.17. Cancer Death Rates per 100,000—Women

Cancer	Asian/Pacific-Islander Women	Non-Hispanic White Women	Asian/Pacific-Islander/ Non-Hispanic White Ratio
All sites	84.6	137.8	0.6
Liver and IBD	5.4	3.6	1.5

Source: NCI, 2021.

Table 34.18 provides the age-adjusted death rates per 100,000 for chronic liver disease and cirrhosis, comparing non-Hispanic Asian and non-Hispanic white populations.[1]

Table 34.18. Age-Adjusted Chronic Liver Disease and Cirrhosis Death Rates per 100,000 (2018)

Sex	Non-Hispanic Asian	Non-Hispanic White	Non-Hispanic Asian/ Non-Hispanic White Ratio
Men	4.6	14.9	0.3
Women	2.4	8.3	0.3
Total	3.4	11.5	0.3

Source: CDC, 2021.

Section 34.4 | **Chronic Liver Disease and Hispanic Americans**

HOW DOES CHRONIC LIVER DISEASE AFFECT HISPANIC AMERICANS?

According to the Centers for Disease Control and Prevention (CDC), chronic liver disease includes health problems that affect the liver over time. The liver is the body's largest internal

[1] Office of Minority Health (OMH), "Chronic Liver Disease and Asian Americans," U.S. Department of Health and Human Services (HHS), 2021. Available online. URL: https://minorityhealth.hhs.gov/chronic-liver-disease-and-asian-americans. Accessed October 1, 2024.

organ. It lies under the ribs on the right side of the abdomen. The liver performs many important functions, including removing waste from the body, such as toxins and medicines, making bile to help digest food, storing sugar that the body uses for energy, and producing new proteins. Liver disease affects the way the liver functions.

Among the Hispanic/Latino population, chronic liver disease is a leading cause of death. While the exact cause is not always known, some cases can be initiated by conditions such as chronic alcoholism, obesity, and exposure to hepatitis B and C viruses.

- In 2019, chronic liver disease was the seventh leading cause of death for all Hispanics and the fourth leading cause of death for Hispanic men aged 45–54.
- Hispanic men and women are 1.5 and 1.6 times more likely to die, respectively, from liver and intrahepatic bile duct (IBD) cancer compared to their non-Hispanic white counterparts.

CANCER RATES (2017–2021)

Table 34.19 provides the age-adjusted cancer incidence rates per 100,000 population for Hispanic (any race) males and non-Hispanic white males.

Table 34.19. Cancer Incidence in Males, Age-Adjusted Rate per 100,000 Population, 2017–2021

Cancer	Hispanic (Any Race) Males	Non-Hispanic White Males	Hispanic (Any Race)/ Non-Hispanic White Ratio
All sites	367.0	510.7	0.7
Liver and IBD	21.5	11.2	1.9

Source: NCI, 2024.

Table 34.20 provides the age-adjusted cancer incidence rates per 100,000 population for Hispanic (any race) females and non-Hispanic white females.

Table 34.20. Cancer Incidence in Females, Age-Adjusted Rate per 100,000 Population, 2017–2021

Cancer	Hispanic (Any Race) Females	Non-Hispanic White Females	Hispanic (Any Race)/ Non-Hispanic White Ratio
All sites	347.8	447.0	0.8
Liver and IBD	9.4	4.3	2.2

Source: NCI, 2024.

DIAGNOSED

Table 34.21 provides the age-adjusted percentage of adults aged 18 and over who have been diagnosed with chronic liver disease.

Table 34.21. Adults Aged 18 and Over Who Have Been Told by a Doctor That They Have Chronic Liver Disease, Age-Adjusted Percentage, 2018

	Population	Non-Hispanic White	Population/Non-Hispanic White Ratio
All Hispanic	2.7	1.6	1.7
Mexican American	3.4	1.6	2.0

Source: CDC, 2020.

DEATH RATES

Table 34.22 provides the age-adjusted cancer mortality rates per 100,000 population for Hispanic (any race) males and non-Hispanic white males.

Table 34.22. Cancer Mortality in Males, Age-Adjusted Rate per 100,000 Population, 2018–2022

Cancer	Hispanic (Any Race) Males	Non-Hispanic White Males	Hispanic (Any Race)/ Non-Hispanic White Ratio
All sites	126.8	179.0	0.7
Liver and IBD	12.6	8.4	1.5

Source: NCI, 2024.

Chronic Liver Disease

Table 34.23 provides the age-adjusted cancer mortality rates per 100,000 population for Hispanic (any race) females and non-Hispanic white females.

Table 34.23. Cancer Mortality in Females, Age-Adjusted Rate per 100,000 Population, 2018–2022

Cancer	Hispanic (Any Race) Females	Non-Hispanic White Females	Hispanic (Any Race)/ Non-Hispanic White Ratio
All sites	93.2	131.0	0.7
Liver and IBD	6.1	3.8	1.6

Source: NCI, 2024.

Table 34.24 provides the age-adjusted mortality rates for chronic liver disease and cirrhosis per 100,000 population, comparing Hispanic and non-Hispanic white populations.[1]

Table 34.24. Chronic Liver Disease and Cirrhosis Mortality, Age-Adjusted Rates per 100,000 Population, 2020

Sex	Hispanic	Non-Hispanic White	Hispanic/Non-Hispanic White Ratio
Male	22.8	18.0	1.3
Female	10.2	10.3	1.0
Both sexes	16.4	14.0	1.2

Source: CDC, 2023.

[1] Office of Minority Health (OMH), "Chronic Liver Disease and Hispanic Americans," U.S. Department of Health and Human Services (HHS), 2021. Available online. URL: https://minorityhealth.hhs.gov/chronic-liver-disease-and-hispanic-americans. Accessed October 1, 2024.

Section 34.5 | Chronic Liver Disease and Native Hawaiian/ Pacific Islanders

HOW DOES CHRONIC LIVER DISEASE AFFECT NATIVE HAWAIIAN/PACIFIC ISLANDERS?

According to the Centers for Disease Control and Prevention (CDC), chronic liver disease includes health problems that affect the liver over time. The liver is the body's largest internal organ. It lies under the ribs on the right side of the abdomen. The liver performs many important functions, including removing waste from the body, such as toxins and medicines, making bile to help digest food, storing sugar that the body uses for energy, and producing new proteins. Liver disease affects the way the liver functions.

- Native Hawaiians and Pacific Islanders were seven times more likely to be diagnosed with chronic liver disease in 2006 compared to non-Hispanic whites.
- American Samoans were eight times more likely to develop liver cancer compared to non-Hispanic whites from 1998 to 2002.

Recently published survey data on this topic from the CDC and the National Cancer Institute (NCI) is limited.

CANCER RATES FOR NATIVE HAWAIIANS/PACIFIC ISLANDERS

Table 34.25 provides liver and intrahepatic bile duct (IBD) cancer incidence rates per 100,000 population for Native Hawaiian, Samoan, and non-Hispanic white men.

Table 34.25. Liver and IBD Cancer Incidence Rates per 100,000—Men (1998–2002)

Native Hawaiian	Samoan	Non-Hispanic White	Native Hawaiian/ Non-Hispanic White Ratio	Samoan/Non-Hispanic White Ratio
16.3	54.5	6.7	2.4	8.1

Source: NCI, 2008.

Chronic Liver Disease

Table 34.26 provides liver and IBD cancer incidence rates per 100,000 population for Native Hawaiian and non-Hispanic white women.

Table 34.26. Liver and IBD Cancer Incidence Rates per 100,000—Women (1998–2002)

Native Hawaiian	Non-Hispanic White	Native Hawaiian/ Non-Hispanic White Ratio
7.7	2.6	3.0

Source: NCI, 2008.

DIAGNOSED

Table 34.27 provides the age-adjusted percentage of adults aged 18 and over diagnosed with chronic liver disease, comparing Native Hawaiian/Pacific-Islander and non-Hispanic white populations.

Table 34.27. Age-Adjusted Percentage of Adults Aged 18 and Over Who Have Been Told by a Doctor That They Have Chronic Liver Disease, 2006

Native Hawaiian/ Pacific Islander	Non-Hispanic White	Native Hawaiian/Pacific-Islander/Non-Hispanic White Ratio
9.7	1.4	7.0

Source: CDC, 2007.

DEATH RATES (2014–2018)

Table 34.28 provides liver and IBD cancer death rates per 100,000 population for Native Hawaiian, Samoan, and non-Hispanic white men.

Table 34.28. Cancer Death Rates per 100,000—Men (1998–2002)

Cancer	Native Hawaiian	Samoan	Non-Hispanic White	Native Hawaiian/ Non-Hispanic White Ratio	Samoan/ Non-Hispanic White Ratio
Live and IBD	11.8	32.9	6.1	1.9	5.4

Source: NCI, 2008.

Table 34.29 provides liver and IBD cancer death rates per 100,000 population for Native Hawaiian, Samoan (data not available), and non-Hispanic white women.

Table 34.29. Cancer Death Rates per 100,000—Women (1998–2002)

Cancer	Native Hawaiian	Samoan	Non-Hispanic White	Native Hawaiian/ Non-Hispanic White Ratio	Samoan/ Non-Hispanic White Ratio
Live and IBD	6.4	—	2.7	2.4	—

Source: NCI, 2008.

Table 34.30 provides the age-adjusted death rates for chronic liver disease and cirrhosis per 100,000 population, comparing non-Hispanic Native Hawaiian/Pacific-Islander and non-Hispanic white populations.[1]

Table 34.30. Age-Adjusted Chronic Liver Disease and Cirrhosis Death Rates per 100,000 (2018)

Sex	Non-Hispanic Native Hawaiian/Pacific Islander	Non-Hispanic White	Non-Hispanic Native Hawaiian/Pacific-Islander/ Non-Hispanic White Ratio
Men	9.9	14.9	0.7
Women	—	8.3	—
Total	7.9	11.5	0.7

Source: CDC, 2021.

[1] Office of Minority Health (OMH), "Chronic Liver Disease and Native Hawaiian/Pacific Islander," U.S. Department of Health and Human Services (HHS), 2021. Available online. URL: https://minorityhealth.hhs.gov/chronic-liver-disease-and-native-hawaiianpacific-islander. Accessed October 1, 2024.

Chapter 35 | **Mental and Behavioral Health**

Chapter Contents

Section 35.1 | **Mental and Behavioral Health and African Americans**

HOW DOES MENTAL AND BEHAVIORAL HEALTH AFFECT AFRICAN-AMERICAN POPULATIONS?

According to the Centers for Disease Control and Prevention (CDC), mental health includes our emotional, psychological, and social well-being. It affects how we think, feel, and act. It also helps determine how we handle stress, relate to others, and make healthy choices. Mental health is important at every stage of life, from childhood and adolescence through adulthood. Behavioral health pertains more to the specific actions people take and how they respond in various scenarios. Behavioral health can be influenced by an individual's mental health.

- Suicide was the third leading cause of death for Black or African-American individuals aged 15–24 years in 2010.
- The death rate from suicide for Black or African-American men was four times greater than for African-American women in 2018.
- The overall suicide rate for Black or African-American individuals was 60 percent lower than that of the non-Hispanic white population in 2018.
- Black females in grades 9–12 were 60 percent more likely to attempt suicide in 2019 compared to non-Hispanic white females of the same age.
- Poverty level affects mental health status. Black or African-American individuals living below the poverty level, compared to those over twice the poverty level, are twice as likely to report serious psychological distress.
- A report from the U.S. Surgeon General found that from 1980 to 1995, the suicide rate among African Americans aged 10–14 years increased by 233 percent, compared to 120 percent of non-Hispanic whites.

MENTAL HEALTH STATUS

Table 35.1 provides the percentage of adults aged 18 and over who experienced serious psychological distress in the past year, comparing non-Hispanic Black and non-Hispanic white populations.

Table 35.1. Serious Psychological Distress in the Past Year among Adults Aged 18 and Over, Percentage, 2019

Non-Hispanic Black	Non-Hispanic White	Non-Hispanic Black/ Non-Hispanic White Ratio
11.9	12.7	0.9

Source: SAMHSA, 2022.

Table 35.2 provides the percentage of adults aged 18 and over who experienced serious psychological distress in the past 30 days, categorized by poverty level and comparing non-Hispanic Black and non-Hispanic white populations.

Table 35.2. Serious Psychological Distress in the Past 30 Days among Adults Aged 18 and Over, Percentage of Poverty Level, 2015–2016

	Non-Hispanic Black	Non-Hispanic White	Non-Hispanic Black/ Non-Hispanic White Ratio
Below 100 percent	7.6	12.1	0.9
100–200 percent	3.9	7.6	0.5
200–400 percent	2.8	3.1	0.9

Source: CDC, 2021.

Table 35.3 provides the percentage of adults aged 18 and over who reported experiencing feelings of sadness, hopelessness, worthlessness, or that everything is an effort all or most of the time.

Table 35.3. Percentage of Population with Feelings of Sadness, Hopelessness, Worthlessness, or That Everything Is an Effort, All or Most of the Time, among Adults Aged 18 and Over, 2018

	Non-Hispanic Black	**Non-Hispanic White**	**Non-Hispanic Black/ Non-Hispanic White Ratio**
Sadness	4.2	2.6	1.6
Hopelessness	1.8	2.2	0.8
Worthlessness	1.8	2.3	0.7
Everything is an effort	11.0	6.6	1.7

Source: CDC, 2021.

Table 35.4 provides the percentage of adults aged 18 and over who experienced serious psychological distress, categorized by sex and comparing non-Hispanic Black and non-Hispanic white populations.

Table 35.4. Percentage of Population with Serious Psychological Distress among Adults Aged 18 and Over, 2018

Sex	**Non-Hispanic Black**	**Non-Hispanic White**	**Non-Hispanic Black/ Non-Hispanic White Ratio**
Men	2.5	2.8	0.9
Women	4.7	4.8	1.0
Total	3.7	3.8	1.0

Source: CDC, 2021.

DEATH RATES

Table 35.5 provides age-adjusted suicide death rates per 100,000 population, comparing non-Hispanic Black and non-Hispanic white populations by sex.

Table 35.5. Age-Adjusted Death Rates for Suicide, by Sex, Race, and Hispanic Origin, 2019

Sex	Non-Hispanic Black	Non-Hispanic White	Non-Hispanic Black/ Non-Hispanic White Ratio
Male	12.7	28.0	0.5
Female	2.9	7.7	0.4
Total	7.5	17.7	0.4

Source: CDC, 2021.

ACCESS TO MENTAL HEALTH SERVICES

Table 35.6 provides the percentage of adults aged 18 and over who received mental health services, comparing non-Hispanic Black and non-Hispanic white populations.[1]

Table 35.6. Percentage of Adults Aged 18 and Over Who Received Mental Health Services in the Past Year, 2020

Non-Hispanic Black	Non-Hispanic White	Non-Hispanic Black/ Non-Hispanic White Ratio
37.1	51.8	0.6

Source: SAMHSA, 2022.

Section 35.2 | Mental and Behavioral Health and American Indians/Alaska Natives

HOW DOES MENTAL AND BEHAVIORAL HEALTH AFFECT AMERICAN INDIANS/ALASKA NATIVES?

According to the Centers for Disease Control and Prevention (CDC), mental health includes our emotional, psychological, and

[1] Office of Minority Health (OMH), "Mental and Behavioral Health—African Americans," U.S. Department of Health and Human Services (HHS), 2021. Available online. URL: https://minorityhealth.hhs.gov/mental-and-behavioral-health-african-americans. Accessed October 1, 2024.

social well-being. It affects how we think, feel, and act. It also helps determine how we handle stress, relate to others, and make healthy choices. Mental health is important at every stage of life, from childhood and adolescence through adulthood. Behavioral health pertains more to the specific actions people take and how they respond in various scenarios. Behavioral health can be influenced by an individual's mental health.

- In 2020, suicide was the second leading cause of death for American Indians/Alaska Natives between the ages of 10 and 34 years.
- American Indians/Alaska Natives are 60 percent more likely to experience the feeling that everything is an effort, all or most of the time, compared to non-Hispanic whites.
- The overall death rate from suicide for American Indian/Alaska Native adults is approximately 20 percent higher compared to the non-Hispanic white population.
- In 2019, adolescent American Indian/Alaska Native females, aged 15–19, had a death rate that was five times higher than non-Hispanic white females in the same age group.
- In 2018, American Indian/Alaska Native males, aged 15–24, had a death rate that was twice that of non-Hispanic white males in the same age group.
- Violent deaths, including unintentional injuries, homicide, and suicide, account for 75 percent of all mortality in the second decade of life for American Indians/Alaska Natives.

MENTAL HEALTH STATUS

Table 35.7 provides the percentage of adults aged 18 and over who experienced serious psychological distress in the past year, comparing American Indian/Alaska Native and non-Hispanic white populations.

Table 35.7. Serious Psychological Distress in the Past Year among Adults Aged 18 and Over, Percentage, 2019

American Indian/ Alaska Native	Non-Hispanic White	American Indian/Alaska Native/ Non-Hispanic White Ratio
11.6	12.7	0.9

Source: SAMHSA, 2020.

Table 35.8 provides the percentage of adults aged 18 and over who reported feelings of sadness, hopelessness, worthlessness, or that everything is an effort all or most of the time, comparing American Indian/Alaska Native and non-Hispanic white populations.

Table 35.8. Percentage of Population with Feelings of Sadness, Hopelessness, Worthlessness, or That Everything Is an Effort, All or Most of the Time, among Adults Aged 18 and Over, 2018

	American Indian/ Alaska Native	Non-Hispanic White	American Indian/ Alaska Native/ Non-Hispanic White Ratio
Sadness	—	2.6	—
Hopelessness	—	2.2	—
Worthlessness	3.4	2.3	1.5
Everything is an effort	10.5	6.6	1.6

Source: CDC, 2021.

Table 35.9 provides the percentage of adults aged 18 and over who experienced serious psychological distress, comparing American Indian/Alaska Native and non-Hispanic white populations.

Table 35.9. Percentage of Population with Serious Psychological Distress among Adults Aged 18 and Over, 2018

	American Indian/ Alaska Native	Non-Hispanic White	American Indian/Alaska Native/ Non-Hispanic White Ratio
Total	4.5	3.8	1.2

Source: CDC, 2021.

DEATH RATES

Table 35.10 provides the age-adjusted suicide death rates per 100,000 population, comparing American Indian/Alaska Native and non-Hispanic white populations by sex.

Table 35.10. Age-Adjusted Death Rates for Suicide, by Sex, Race and Hispanic Origin, 2018

Sex	American Indian/ Alaska Native	Non-Hispanic White	American Indian/ Alaska Native/ Non-Hispanic White Ratio
Male	33.6	28.6	1.2
Female	11.1	8.0	1.4
Total	22.3	18.1	1.2

Source: CDC, 2021.

ACCESS TO HEALTH CARE

Table 35.11 provides the percentage of adults aged 18 and over who received mental health services in the past year, comparing American Indian/Alaska Native and non-Hispanic white populations.[1]

Table 35.11. Percentage of Adults Aged 18 and Over Who Received Mental Health Services in the Past Year, 2019

American Indian/ Alaska Native	Non-Hispanic White	American Indian/ Alaska Native/ Non-Hispanic White Ratio
13.9	19.8	0.7

Source: SAMHSA, 2020.

[1] Office of Minority Health (OMH), "Mental and Behavioral Health—American Indians/Alaska Natives," U.S. Department of Health and Human Services (HHS), 2021. Available online. URL: https://minorityhealth.hhs.gov/mental-and-behavioral-health-american-indiansalaska-natives. Accessed October 2, 2024.

Section 35.3 | Mental and Behavioral Health and Asian Americans

HOW DOES MENTAL AND BEHAVIORAL HEALTH AFFECT ASIAN AMERICANS?

According to the Centers for Disease Control and Prevention (CDC), mental health includes our emotional, psychological, and social well-being. It affects how we think, feel, and act. It also helps determine how we handle stress, relate to others, and make healthy choices. Mental health is important at every stage of life, from childhood and adolescence through adulthood. Behavioral health pertains more to the specific actions people take and how they respond in various scenarios. Behavioral health can be influenced by an individual's mental health.

- Suicide was the leading cause of death for Asian/Pacific Islanders aged 15–24 in 2019.
- Asian-American males in grades 9–12 were 30 percent more likely to consider attempting suicide compared to non-Hispanic white male students in the same year.
- In 2018, Asians were 60 percent less likely to have received mental health treatment compared to non-Hispanic whites.
- Southeast Asian refugees are at risk for posttraumatic stress disorder (PTSD) associated with trauma experienced before and after immigration to the United States. One study found that 70 percent of Southeast Asian refugees receiving mental health care were diagnosed with PTSD.
- The overall suicide rate for Asians is less than half that of the non-Hispanic white population.

MENTAL HEALTH STATUS

Table 35.12 provides the percentage of adults aged 18 and over who experienced serious psychological distress in the past year, comparing Asian and non-Hispanic white populations.

Table 35.12. Serious Psychological Distress in the Past Year among Adults Aged 18 and Over, Percentage, 2019

Asian	Non-Hispanic White	Asian/Non-Hispanic White Ratio
9.0	12.7	0.6

Source: SAMHSA, 2020.

Table 35.13 provides the percentage of adults aged 18 and over who reported feelings of sadness, hopelessness, worthlessness, or that everything is an effort all of the time, comparing Asian and non-Hispanic white populations.

Table 35.13. Percentage of Population with Feelings of Sadness, Hopelessness, Worthlessness, or That Everything Is an Effort, All of the Time, among Adults Aged 18 and Over, 2018

	Asian	Non-Hispanic White	Asian/Non-Hispanic White Ratio
Sadness	1.6	2.6	0.7
Hopelessness	1.4	2.2	0.6
Worthlessness	1.9	2.3	0.4
Everything is an effort	6.7	6.6	0.7

Source: CDC, 2021.

Table 35.14 provides the percentage of adults aged 18 and over who experienced serious psychological distress, comparing Asian and non-Hispanic white populations.

Table 35.14. Percentage of Population with Serious Psychological Distress among Adults Aged 18 and Over, 2018

Asian	Non-Hispanic White	Asian/Non-Hispanic White Ratio
2.1	3.8	0.0

Source: CDC, 2021.

Table 35.15 provides the age-adjusted percentage distributions of adults aged 18 and over who experienced serious psychological distress most or all of the time, comparing various Asian subgroups with the overall Asian and non-Hispanic white populations.

Table 35.15. Age-Adjusted Percentage Distributions of Adults Aged 18 and Over, with Serious Psychological Distress, Most or All of the Time, 2004–2006

Population	Serious Distress	Ratio/All Asian Population	Ratio/Whites
All whites	2.9	—	—
All Asians	1.9	—	1.7
Chinese	1.6	0.8	0.6
Filipino	2.5	1.3	0.9
Asian Indian	1.4	0.7	0.5
Japanese	1.1	0.6	0.4
Vietnamese	2.5	1.3	0.9
Korean	1.3	0.7	0.4
Other Asian and NHOPI	2.6	1.4	0.9

Source: CDC, 2008.

DEATH RATES

Table 35.16 provides the age-adjusted suicide death rates per 100,000 population, comparing Asian and non-Hispanic white populations by sex.

Table 35.16. Age-Adjusted Death Rates for Suicide, by Sex, Race and Hispanic Origin, 2018

Sex	Asian	Non-Hispanic White	Asian/Non-Hispanic White Ratio
Male	10.0	28.6	0.4
Female	3.8	8.0	0.5
Total	6.7	18.1	0.4

Source: CDC, 2021.

ACCESS TO HEALTH CARE

Table 35.17 provides the percentage of adults aged 18 and over who received mental health services in the past year, comparing Asian and non-Hispanic white populations.[1]

Table 35.17. Percentage of Adults Aged 18 and Over Who Received Mental Health Services in the Past Year, 2019

Asian	Non-Hispanic White	Asian/Non-Hispanic White Ratio
7.0	19.8	0.3

Source: SAMHSA, 2020.

Section 35.4 | Mental and Behavioral Health and Hispanic Americans

HOW DOES MENTAL AND BEHAVIORAL HEALTH AFFECT HISPANIC AMERICANS?

According to the Centers for Disease Control and Prevention (CDC), mental health includes our emotional, psychological, and social well-being. It affects how we think, feel, and act. It also helps determine how we handle stress, relate to others, and make healthy choices. Mental health is important at every stage of life, from childhood and adolescence through adulthood. Behavioral health pertains more to the specific actions people take and how they respond in various scenarios. Behavioral health can be influenced by an individual's mental health.

- The death rate from suicide for Hispanic males was 4.4 times higher than that for Hispanic women in 2020.
- In that same year, the suicide death rate for Hispanics was less than half the rate for non-Hispanic whites.

[1] Office of Minority Health (OMH), "Mental and Behavioral Health—Asian Americans," U.S. Department of Health and Human Services (HHS), 2021. Available online. URL: https://minorityhealth.hhs.gov/mental-and-behavioral-health-asian-americans. Accessed October 1, 2024.

- Additionally, in 2022, Hispanic adults were 60 percent less likely to have received mental health treatment compared to non-Hispanic white adults.

MENTAL HEALTH STATUS

Table 35.18 provides the percentage of adults aged 18 and over who experienced serious psychological distress in the past year, comparing Hispanic and non-Hispanic white populations.

Table 35.18. Serious Psychological Distress in the Past Year among Adults Aged 18 and Over, Percentage, 2022

Hispanic	Non-Hispanic White	Hispanic/Non-Hispanic White Ratio
14.2	15.0	0.9

Source: SAMHSA, 2023.

Table 35.19 provides the percentage of adults aged 18 and over who experienced serious psychological distress in the past 30 days, categorized by poverty level and comparing Hispanic and non-Hispanic white populations.

Table 35.19. Serious Psychological Distress in the Past 30 Days among Adults Aged 18 and Over, Percentage of Poverty Level, 2015–2016

	Hispanic	Non-Hispanic White	Hispanic/Non-Hispanic White Ratio
Below 100 percent	6.8	12.1	0.6
100–200 percent	4.1	7.6	0.5
200–400 percent	2.6	3.1	0.8

Source: CDC, 2019.

Table 35.20 provides the percentage of adults aged 18 and over who reported feelings of sadness, hopelessness, worthlessness, or that everything is an effort all or most of the time, comparing Hispanic and non-Hispanic white populations.

Table 35.20. Feelings of Sadness, Hopelessness, Worthlessness, or That Everything Is an Effort, All or Most of the Time, among Adults Aged 18 and Over, 2018

	Hispanic	Non-Hispanic White	Hispanic/Non-Hispanic White Ratio
Sadness	3.9	2.7	1.4
Hopelessness	3.2	2.2	1.5
Worthlessness	2.4	2.3	1.0
Everything is an effort	7.3	6.5	1.1

Source: CDC, 2021.

Table 35.21 provides the percentage of adults aged 18 and over who experienced serious psychological distress, comparing Hispanic and non-Hispanic white populations by sex.

Table 35.21. Serious Psychological Distress among Adults Aged 18 and Over, Percentage, 2018

Sex	Hispanic	Non-Hispanic White	Hispanic/Non-Hispanic White Ratio
Male	3.5	2.7	1.3
Female	5.4	4.7	1.1
Total	4.4	3.7	1.2

Source: CDC, 2021.

DEATH RATES

Table 35.22 provides the age-adjusted suicide death rates per 100,000 population, comparing Hispanic and non-Hispanic white populations by sex.

Table 35.22. Age-Adjusted Death Rates for Suicide by Sex, Race, and Hispanic Origin, 2020

Sex	Hispanic	Non-Hispanic White	Hispanic/Non-Hispanic White Ratio
Male	12.3	27.2	0.5
Female	2.8	6.9	0.4
Total	7.5	16.9	0.4

Source: CDC, 2023.

ACCESS TO HEALTH CARE

Table 35.23 provides the percentage of adults aged 18 and over who received mental health treatment in the past year, comparing Hispanic and non-Hispanic white populations.[1]

Table 35.23. Adults Aged 18 and Over Who Received Mental Health Treatment in the Past Year, Percentage, 2022

Hispanic	Non-Hispanic White	Hispanic/Non-Hispanic White Ratio
14.6	25.9	0.6

Source: SAMHSA, 2023.

Section 35.5 | Mental and Behavioral Health and Native Hawaiian/Pacific Islanders

HOW DOES MENTAL AND BEHAVIORAL HEALTH AFFECT NATIVE HAWAIIAN/PACIFIC ISLANDERS?

According to the Centers for Disease Control and Prevention (CDC), mental health includes our emotional, psychological, and social well-being. It affects how we think, feel, and act. It also helps determine how we handle stress, relate to others, and make healthy choices. Mental health is important at every stage of life, from childhood and adolescence through adulthood. Behavioral health pertains more to the specific actions people take and how they respond in various scenarios. Behavioral health can be influenced by an individual's mental health.

- In 2019, suicide was the leading cause of death for Native Hawaiians/Pacific Islanders aged 15–24.
- In 2019, Native Hawaiians/Pacific Islanders were three times less likely to receive mental health services or prescription medications for mental health treatment compared to non-Hispanic whites.

[1] Office of Minority Health (OMH), "Mental and Behavioral Health—Hispanics," U.S. Department of Health and Human Services (HHS), 2021. Available online. URL: https://minorityhealth.hhs.gov/mental-and-behavioral-health-hispanics. Accessed October 2, 2024.

MENTAL HEALTH STATUS

Table 35.24 provides the percentage of adults aged 18 and over who experienced serious psychological distress in the past year, comparing Native Hawaiian/Pacific-Islander and non-Hispanic white populations.

Table 35.24. Serious Psychological Distress in the Past Year among Adults Aged 18 and Over, Percentage, 2019

Native Hawaiian/ Pacific Islander	Non-Hispanic White	Native Hawaiian/Pacific-Islander/ Non-Hispanic White Ratio
10.1	12.7	0.8

Source: SAMHSA, 2020.

Table 35.25 provides the percentage of adults aged 18 and over who had a major depressive episode in the past year, comparing Native Hawaiian/Pacific-Islander and non-Hispanic white populations.

Table 35.25. Adults Aged 18 and Over with Major Depressive Episode in the Past Year, 2019

Native Hawaiian/ Pacific Islander	Non-Hispanic White	Native Hawaiian/Pacific-Islander/ Non-Hispanic White Ratio
3.5	8.5	0.4

Source: SAMHSA, 2020.

Table 35.26 provides the percentage of adults aged 18 and over who experienced any mental illness in the past year, comparing Native Hawaiian/Pacific-Islander and non-Hispanic white populations.

Table 35.26. Adults Aged 18 and Over with Any Mental Illness in the Past Year, 2019

Native Hawaiian/ Pacific Islander	Non-Hispanic White	Native Hawaiian/Pacific-Islander/ Non-Hispanic White Ratio
16.6	22.2	0.7

Source: SAMHSA, 2020.

DEATH RATES

Table 35.27 provides the age-adjusted suicide death rates per 100,000 population, comparing Native Hawaiian/Pacific-Islander and non-Hispanic white populations by sex.

Table 35.27. Age-Adjusted Death Rates for Suicide, by Sex, Race and Hispanic Origin, 2018

Sex	Native Hawaiian/ Pacific Islander	Non-Hispanic White	Native Hawaiian/Pacific-Islander/Non-Hispanic White Ratio
Male	19.8	28.6	0.7
Female	—	8.0	—
Total	11.9	18.1	0.7

Source: CDC, 2021.

ACCESS TO HEALTH CARE

Table 35.28 provides the percentage of adults aged 18 and over who received mental health services in the past year, comparing Native Hawaiian/Pacific-Islander and non-Hispanic white populations.[1]

Table 35.28. Percentage of Adults Aged 18 and Over Who Received Mental Health Services in the Past Year, 2019

Native Hawaiian/ Pacific Islander	Non-Hispanic White	Native Hawaiian/Pacific-Islander/ Non-Hispanic White Ratio
6.1	19.8	0.3

Source: SAMHSA, 2020.

[1] Office of Minority Health (OMH), "Mental and Behavioral Health—Native Hawaiians/Pacific Islanders," U.S. Department of Health and Human Services (HHS), 2021. Available online. URL: https://minorityhealth.hhs.gov/mental-and-behavioral-health-native-hawaiianspacific-islanders. Accessed October 2, 2024.

Part 6 | Strategies for Health-Care Improvement and Equity

Chapter 36 | Expanding Health Insurance Access and Benefits through the Affordable Care Act

Health insurance is critical to providing affordable access to medical care and improving health and well-being. It offers individuals financial protection from out-of-pocket spending for needed health care and is associated with improved health outcomes, lower death rates, and increased productivity. Health coverage provided by or subsidized by the federal government and states acts as an important component of the social safety net and ensures that low-income individuals and older adults can obtain the care they need in an affordable, accessible manner.

THE AFFORDABLE CARE ACT

The Patient Protection and Affordable Care Act (ACA), which was enacted in 2010 to bolster this health-care safety net, was the most significant health policy legislation since the establishment of Medicare and Medicaid in 1965. By 2015, the year after the main coverage provisions of the law went into effect, over 90 percent of all Americans benefited from health insurance coverage.

After enrollment stagnated from 2016 to 2021, the ACA Marketplaces have experienced double-digit growth in enrollment each year since 2021. As a result of legislation enacted in 2021 and 2022, consumers' share of Marketplace premiums has fallen, with the majority of HealthCare.gov enrollees being able to choose a zero-premium plan, and enrollment has expanded by more than

77 percent to over 21 million Americans. Enrollment in Medicaid and the Children's Health Insurance Program (CHIP) has also grown as four additional states (North Carolina, Missouri, South Dakota, and Oklahoma) adopted the ACA Medicaid expansion in 2021. New continuous eligibility rules make it easier for children and new mothers to retain Medicaid coverage.

RESEARCH ON THE BENEFITS OF HEALTH INSURANCE

The design of the ACA was informed by a large academic literature on the economics of health care and health insurance, including numerous studies showing that insurance coverage leads to better access to and utilization of care. The ACA coverage expansions, in turn, have fueled a dramatic growth of studies that have helped us understand the effects of health insurance on both health outcomes and other outcomes related to individual and societal well-being. This research finds the effects of health insurance coverage on improved access to care, increased utilization of preventive care, better health outcomes, financial benefits, and reduced income inequality.

IMPROVEMENTS IN ACCESS TO CARE

The effects of increased health insurance coverage on access were quickly evident following the implementation of the ACA's key coverage provisions. Studies documented improvements in rates of self-reported access, including having a primary care physician, having easy access to medicine, the ability to afford care, and the percentage of days with activities limited by health. Measures of access and affordability, such as having a routine checkup and fewer problems accessing care, improved for adults at all income levels and regardless of state expansion status, though some effects, such as reductions in problems paying family medical bills, unmet needs for care because of cost, and not having a usual source of care, were more pronounced for lower income groups. As disparities in health insurance coverage related to race and ethnicity decreased, so too did disparities in access to care.

INCREASED UTILIZATION OF PREVENTIVE SERVICES

Increases in coverage and access lead to increased utilization of care and improved health outcomes. Since the enactment of the ACA, studies have found increased use of cancer screening, human papillomavirus (HPV) vaccination completion rates, influenza vaccinations, Medicare wellness visits, contraception usage, and blood pressure and cholesterol screenings. Studies have also shown increased utilization of prescription drug treatments, with individuals who gained insurance coverage through Medicaid or private insurance filling more prescriptions and having lower out-of-pocket spending on prescriptions.

Improved access to preventive services leads to more timely and appropriate treatment of both acute and chronic conditions. Studies have linked insurance expansions under the ACA to increases in early-stage cancer diagnosis, which is associated with:

- better cancer outcomes
- improved blood pressure and glucose control
- reductions in the probability of pre-term birth

FINANCIAL BENEFITS OF HEALTH INSURANCE COVERAGE

Research on the ACA shows that in addition to these health benefits, health insurance coverage produces substantial financial benefits to both patients and providers. ACA Marketplace subsidies were found to reduce consumer bankruptcies, severe auto delinquency, and third-party collections, while Medicaid expansions were associated with a decrease in medical debt, the number of unpaid bills, the amount of unpaid balances in collections, and the use of payday loans, as well as an increase in financial satisfaction. Research documents a decline in home evictions in Medicaid expansion states as compared to non-expansion states, despite comparable rates prior to expansion. Further, expansion has been associated with a reduction in the poverty rate, with one study estimating that nearly 700,000 fewer Americans were living in poverty as a result of Medicaid expansion.

FUTURE OPPORTUNITIES FOR COVERAGE EXPANSION

The insurance coverage of low-income Americans could be increased further if every state implemented the ACA Medicaid expansion. It is estimated that if the 10 states that have not yet expanded did so, 2.3 million people would gain access to coverage. As with earlier expansions, the coverage gains would be greater for Blacks and Latinos, causing coverage disparities to decrease even more. The evidence developed over the past decade and more shows that coverage gains will translate to improved health and financial well-being for millions of Americans, providing benefits to those who are newly covered, as well as broader financial and societal benefits.[1]

[1] Office of the Assistant Secretary for Planning and Evaluation (ASPE), "Improving Access to Affordable and Equitable Health Coverage: A Review from 2010 to 2024," U.S. Department of Health and Human Services (HHS), June 7, 2024. Available online. URL: https://aspe.hhs.gov/sites/default/files/documents/9376755db2480ad7288aaa5ec38f3d8c/improving-access-to-coverage.pdf. Accessed September 30, 2024.

Chapter 37 | Improving Health Literacy for Better Health Outcomes

The definition of health literacy was updated in August 2020 with the release of the U.S. government's Healthy People 2030 initiative (https://health.gov/healthypeople/priority-areas/health-literacy-healthy-people-2030). The update addresses personal health literacy and organizational health literacy and provides the following definitions:

- "Personal health literacy" is the degree to which people have the ability to find, understand, and use information and services to inform health-related decisions and actions for themselves and others.
- "Organizational health literacy" is the degree to which organizations equitably enable people to find, understand, and use information and services to inform health-related decisions and actions for themselves and others.

These definitions differ from the health literacy definition used in Healthy People 2010 and Healthy People 2020: "the degree to which people have the capacity to obtain, process, and understand basic health information and services needed to make appropriate health decisions."

The new definitions:

- Emphasize people's ability to use health information rather than just understand it.
- Focus on the ability to make "well-informed" decisions rather than "appropriate" ones.
- Acknowledge that organizations have a responsibility to address health literacy.
- Incorporate a public health perspective.

From a public health perspective, the organizational definition acknowledges that health literacy is connected to health equity. "Health equity" is the attainment of the highest level of health for all people. Health equity is achieved when everyone has the opportunity to be as healthy as possible.

WHY IS HEALTH LITERACY IMPORTANT?

Using health literacy best practices can build trust and advance health equity. Trust is an important part of a person's willingness to engage in care and behaviors that promote health. In 2023, the National Academies of Science, Engineering, and Medicine published proceedings from three workshops in a series titled *The Roles of Trust and Health Literacy in Achieving Health Equity*. Panelists discussed the relationship between health literacy and trust in clinical settings, public health institutions, and community settings. Key recommendations included:

- using plain language
- using the audience's preferred language and communication channels
- using culturally and linguistically appropriate language

HEALTH LITERACY AFFECTS EVERYONE

Health literacy is important for everyone because, at some point in their lives, everyone needs to be able to find, understand, and use health information and services.

Taking care of health is part of everyday life, not just when visiting a doctor, clinic, or hospital. Health literacy can help prevent health problems, protect health, and better manage health problems when they arise.

Even people who read well and are comfortable using numbers can face health literacy issues in certain situations, including the following:

- They are not familiar with medical terms or how their bodies work.
- They have to interpret statistics and evaluate risks and benefits that affect their health and safety.
- They are diagnosed with a serious illness and are scared and confused.

- They have health conditions that require complicated self-care.
- They are voting on an issue affecting the community's health and relying on unfamiliar technical information.

WHY DO WE HAVE A HEALTH LITERACY PROBLEM?

When organizations or individuals create and provide health information that is too difficult to understand, a health literacy problem is created. Expecting people to navigate health services with many unfamiliar, confusing, or conflicting steps also creates a health literacy problem.

HOW CAN WE HELP PEOPLE NOW?

We can help people use the health literacy skills they have in several ways, including the following:

- Create and provide information and services that people can understand and use most effectively with their existing skills.
- Work with educators and others to help people become more familiar with health information and services, and to build their health literacy skills over time.
- Build our own skills as communicators of health information.
- Work with trusted messengers to share information. In many communities, faith leaders and community health workers (also known as "promotores") serve as trusted messengers.
- Build health-literate organizations.
- Consider the cultural and linguistic norms, environment, and history of the intended audience when developing information and messages.
- Use certified translators and interpreters who can adapt to the audience's language preferences, communication expectations, and health literacy skills.[1]

[1] "What Is Health Literacy?" Centers for Disease Control and Prevention (CDC), October 26, 2024. Available online. URL: www.cdc.gov/health-literacy/php/about. Accessed November 2, 2024.

WHAT THE RESEARCH SHOWS

Health literacy can lead to numerous benefits, including the following:

- making more people seek out preventive health care
- improving health outcomes
- decreasing unnecessary emergency room visits
- lowering preventable hospital stays and readmissions
- reducing the number of dosing errors
- helping patients better manage chronic conditions, such as diabetes, high blood pressure, and HIV/AIDS
- improving quality of care
- increasing patient satisfaction

WAYS TO IMPROVE HEALTH LITERACY

Organizations can improve communication and accessibility by implementing the following strategies:

- Create user-friendly systems:
  - patient portals
  - telephone systems
  - forms
- Hire personnel to enhance language accessibility:
  - staff who speak two or more languages
  - interpreters for patients who do not speak English
- Pre-test materials with patients:
  - signs and directions posted in health-care facilities
  - health information that patients can easily read and understand
  - forms and materials in languages other than English
- Provide clear directions for taking medication.

Health-care professionals can take several actions to enhance patient communication, including the following:

- Assume that every patient may not understand you.
- Keep language free of jargon, speak slowly, and use short sentences.
- Use materials that aid learning, such as videos, models, and pictures.

- Apply the Teach-Back method (www.ahrq.gov/patient-safety/reports/engage/teachback.html). Ask patients to:
  - Explain instructions in their own words.
  - Show how they will take their medicine.
- Ask open-ended questions that begin with "How" and "Why."
- Listen to patients' stories without interrupting for a full minute.
- Expect that patients will have questions and be ready to answer them.
- Tell patients only what they need to know—emphasize and repeat the most important points.
- Offer to help complete forms.[2]

[2] "Addressing Health Literacy," Health Resources and Services Administration (HRSA), June 2024. Available online. URL: www.hrsa.gov/about/organization/bureaus/ohe/health-literacy. Accessed September 30, 2024.

Chapter 38 | Strategies for Offering Diverse and Nutritious Foods

Millions of people obtain their food and beverages from worksites or public facilities every day. Implementing food service guidelines in these settings can set a positive example for employees, visitors, community members, and employers from other institutions. Changes in the types of food and beverages available in these environments can enhance the diets of individuals who eat there and contribute to their overall health and wellness.

WHAT ARE CULTURALLY PREFERRED FOODS?

"Culturally preferred foods" describe safe and nutritious foods that meet the diverse tastes and needs of customers based on their cultural identity. For example, people who identify with Muslim or Jewish religious traditions may want foods that are halal or kosher, respectively.

"Culture" can be defined by membership, such as racial, ethnic, linguistic, or geographic groups. Culture may also be a collection of a specific group's beliefs, values, customs, ways of thinking, communication, and behaviors.

WHY ARE CULTURALLY PREFERRED FOODS IMPORTANT?

Offering affordable, culturally preferred food options that align with the *Dietary Guidelines for Americans* (https://health.gov/our-work/nutrition-physical-activity/dietary-guidelines) allows customers to choose foods that meet their needs. Serving culturally preferred food options expands opportunities for customers to select familiar and healthier foods they enjoy. Improved diet quality may positively influence customers' health. Additionally, other customers may learn about and enjoy different cuisines.

WHAT INFLUENCES CUSTOMER FOOD CHOICES?

Beyond cultural preferences, customers choose foods for a variety of reasons, including:

- price, convenience, and taste
- agricultural growing techniques, such as organic farming
- sourcing of products, such as local or regional foods
- food preparation methods, including the use of specific ingredients
- new foods or cuisines
- foods that help prevent or manage chronic health conditions
- food allergies or intolerances

HOW DO I GET SUPPORT FOR CULTURALLY PREFERRED FOODS?

Draw on the expertise of your food service guidelines team, including food service vendors and staff, organizational leadership, and worksite wellness staff. Food service vendors and staff may ensure buy-in and feasibility for including diverse food offerings.

If your food service guidelines team does not already represent the diversity of your customers, consider how to include these perspectives. This is a critical step. However, remember that one person's opinions do not necessarily represent an entire culture.

Discuss with your food service guidelines team the importance of adding culturally diverse foods in various venues, such as cafeterias and vending machines. With your team, you may take the following actions:

- Develop a plan for incorporating culturally preferred foods into food service guidelines.
- Collect ideas and feedback on culturally preferred foods from food service employees and their customers via surveys, interviews, and focus groups.

- Collaborate with food vendors to improve offerings of culturally preferred nutritious options based on customer feedback.

HOW DO I IDENTIFY CULTURALLY PREFERRED FOODS?

Gather Preliminary Information about the Customer Base

Conduct a comprehensive baseline assessment to identify your customers' cultural backgrounds. The human resources department may be able to share some sociodemographic characteristics of customers at the workplace. Next, work with your food service guidelines team to carry out the appropriate qualitative assessments of your customers' food preferences.

Depending on your setting and capacity, you may conduct observational assessments, surveys, informal interviews, and focus groups with customers from diverse cultures. These assessments can reveal customers' perceptions of cultural food offerings and food preferences. Assessments can also identify key facilitators and barriers to offering culturally preferred food options in your setting.

Consider gathering data from food service managers and potential new customers, such as employees who do not currently frequent the food venue.

Assessments can be conducted routinely, as needed. Work with the food service vendor to avoid duplication of effort. Food vendors may already conduct assessments as part of their contractual scope of work.

Develop and Conduct a Customer Survey

Define the goal of your assessment with your food service guidelines team before determining survey questions for your assessment. For example, your primary goal may be to identify top cultural foods enjoyed by your customers to encourage vendors and food service staff to add them to the menu rotations.

Ensure that your questions lead to attaining your goal. Questions can be multiple-choice, scaled (such as Likert), open-ended, qualitative, quantitative, or a combination. Work with your food service guidelines team to identify the appropriate dissemination plan. You may collect surveys using pen and paper or a web-based platform.

If using a web-based platform, consider including a quick response (QR) code for customer convenience.

Consider asking customers questions about cultural foods:

- types of foods embraced by their culture
- cultural habits and traditions, such as religious observances and holidays, that are related to food
- preference for eating foods of their culture when away from home versus foods typically served in food service settings
- facilitators to cultural food purchases, such as visual appeal, prominent display, or low cost
- barriers to cultural food purchases, such as lack of authenticity or variety or not representing customers' cultures
- how often customers eat at the setting and if they would eat there more frequently if culturally desired foods were served

Consider asking customers questions about foods in general:

- use of food to prevent or manage chronic health conditions
- recommendations for improvements to food offerings
- preferences for specialized items to eat food with, such as chopsticks or injera (flat spongy bread made of fermented teff flour)
- favorite items on the current menu

Assess the Current Menu

Examine your setting's menu cycles to determine whether the foods offered represent customers' views and cultures. This will allow you to identify opportunities for improvement.

How Do I Tell Vendors about Adding Cultural Foods to Menus?

If your food vendors are not bound by contract to add culturally diverse foods, ask them if it would be feasible to do so. Any changes must be within the scope of their contract and budget without incurring additional costs.

Consider asking the food vendor questions about the following:

- willingness to offer culturally preferred foods and promote new menu items
- cost-effectiveness of sourcing ingredients
- ability to offer culturally preferred foods that also meet nutrition standards as outlined in the *Dietary Guidelines for Americans*
- whether specialized kitchen equipment might be needed
- knowledge and experience in cooking diverse cuisines and types of foods that would be profitable for vendors
- how often to introduce new or seasonal recipes to the menu rotation
- willingness to offer specific dishes tied to religious observances

If you include sourcing culturally diverse foods in your vendor contracts, the vendor may assess progress voluntarily or as the contract stipulates. Otherwise, consider conducting and sharing assessment findings with your food vendor.

HOW CAN CONTRACTS AND POLICIES HELP?

To ensure cultural food goals are met, consider adding a cultural food standard to your organization's food service guidelines policy. It could state something like, "All onsite food vendors are encouraged to offer a variety of foods related to the cultural heritages of customers and meet the *Dietary Guidelines for Americans*."

Alternatively, your organization could solicit food vendors willing to assess customers' cultural food preferences and include cultural foods in the menu cycles. This can be done via the Request for Proposals (RFP) process. Review bids and select a qualified vendor. Then ensure all cultural food standards are stipulated in the final contract language and the vendor's scope of work.[1]

[1] "Consider Cultural Food Preferences: FAQ," Centers for Disease Control and Prevention (CDC), March 29, 2024. Available online. URL: www.cdc.gov/food-service-guidelines-toolkit/php/strategize-act/cultural-food-preferences.html. Accessed September 30, 2024.

Chapter 39 | Strategies for Enhancing Food Accessibility and Nutrition Security

FOOD ACCESSIBILITY, INSECURITY, AND HEALTH OUTCOMES

Having access to nutritious food is a basic human need.

Food security means having access to enough food for an active, healthy life. Nutrition security means consistent access, availability, and affordability of foods and beverages that promote well-being, prevent disease, and, if needed, treat disease.

On the other hand, food and nutrition insecurity is a major public health concern characterized by limited or uncertain access to adequate and affordable nutritious foods at the individual, household, and neighborhood levels.

Food insecurity and limited access to affordable, nutritious food increase risks for chronic health conditions, including diabetes, obesity, and heart disease. In 2020, nearly 15 percent of U.S. households faced food insecurity, unable to access enough food for healthy living. In nearly half of these households, children were also food insecure, which has implications for human development and school experience.

Food insecurity disproportionately affects individuals from racial and ethnic minority and socioeconomically disadvantaged populations:

- 20 percent of Black/African-American households were food insecure at some point in 2021, compared to 16 percent of Hispanic/Latino households and 7 percent of white households.

- Food insecurity for U.S. Hispanic/Latino adults differs by origin. Although current national data is not available, from 2011 to 2014, food insecurity was highest among those identifying as Puerto Rican (25.3%), followed by those from Mexico (20.8%), Central and South America (20.7%), and Cuba (12.1%).

In the past 20 years, American Indian/Alaskan Native (AI/AN) households have been at least twice as likely to experience food insecurity compared to white households, often exceeding rates of 25 percent across different regions and AI/AN communities. Native Hawaiian and Pacific Islander (NHPI) adults also experience a high prevalence of food insecurity (20.5%) and have significantly higher odds of experiencing low and very low food security compared to white households. While national data on specific Asian-American national origin populations is not readily available, among Asian Americans living in California from 2001 to 2012, food insecurity was highest among Vietnamese households (16.4%), followed by Filipino (8.3%), Chinese (7.6%), Korean (6.7%), South Asian (3.14%), and Japanese households (2.3%), highlighting considerable variation across Asian-American communities.

Food insecurity is inextricably linked to poverty, with 35.3 percent of households with incomes below the federal poverty line being food insecure. Although national trends in food insecurity do not capture the full effect of the coronavirus 2019 (COVID-19) pandemic, it is likely that food insecurity has increased and that racial and ethnic disparities in experiences of food insecurity could worsen.

SOCIAL DETERMINANTS OF HEALTH

Healthy food accessibility and insecurity are social determinants of health. Food and nutrition insecurity are predominantly influenced by the local environment, including neighborhood infrastructure, accessibility, and affordability barriers. Access to grocery stores that carry healthy food options (such as fresh fruit, vegetables, low-fat fish, and poultry) is not equitably distributed across residential and regional areas in the United States.

Areas that lack access to affordable, healthy foods are known as "food deserts." Food deserts are:

- found in urban or suburban neighborhoods that lack grocery stores (supermarkets or small grocery stores) offering healthy food options
- located in rural areas and neighborhoods where the nearest grocery stores are too far away to be convenient or accessible
- more prevalent in neighborhoods comprised of a majority of racial or ethnic minority residents or in rural AI/AN communities
- more likely found in areas with a higher percentage of residents experiencing poverty

Urban, suburban, and rural areas can also be overwhelmed with stores that sell unhealthy, calorie-dense, and inexpensive junk foods, including soda, snacks, and other high-sugar foods. This is known as a "food swamp." Food swamps are characterized by:

- reducing access to nutritional foods while providing easier access to unhealthy options
- being a predictor of obesity, particularly in communities where residents have limited access to personal or public transportation and experience significant income inequality

ADDRESSING FOOD INSECURITY

Reducing food and nutrition insecurity in the United States will require a multifaceted approach that considers, among other possibilities:

- Strategies that engage communities in local health programs, such as recruiting community partners to assist in addressing gaps between food access and intake.
- Interventions that utilize federal food and nutritional supplemental programs, including the Supplemental Nutrition Assistance Program (SNAP) and the Special Supplemental Nutrition Program for Women, Infants, and Children (WIC).

- Leveraging local and federal policies targeting food insecurity, such as retail store interventions where healthy food placement, promotion, and pricing influence healthier choices; implementing sweetened beverage taxes to reduce consumer purchase appeal; and imposing junk food taxes balanced with the removal of taxes on water and fruits and vegetables.[1]

[1] "Food Accessibility, Insecurity and Health Outcomes," National Institute on Minority Health and Health Disparities (NIMHD), July 3, 2024. Available online. URL: www.nimhd.nih.gov/resources/understanding-health-disparities/food-accessibility-insecurity-and-health-outcomes.html. Accessed September 25, 2024.

Chapter 40 | Addressing Tobacco-Related Disparities

Although cigarette smoking has decreased substantially in the United States over the past several decades, declines in prevalence have been slower for some communities. Smoking disparities remain unchanged or have increased for several groups who are targeted by the tobacco industry. Many racial and ethnic minority groups smoke at higher rates than the national average, as do people who identify as belonging to sexual and gender minority groups and those with lower socioeconomic status. At the same time, some subpopulations are at or approaching endgame levels of cigarette use (less than 5%). For example, only 4.1 percent of those with a graduate degree report current cigarette use compared with 23.1 percent of those with less than a high school diploma. Further efforts are needed to achieve low smoking prevalence across all subpopulations.

RISE OF ALTERNATIVE TOBACCO PRODUCTS

Cigarettes remain both the most deadly and commonly used commercial tobacco product; however, many other products (e.g., e-cigarettes, cigars) have gained in popularity. Promotion by the tobacco industry has successfully led to increases in the use of some tobacco products. For instance, e-cigarette use has increased dramatically among youth and young adults in recent years, and the use of cigars has grown in the past two decades among non-Hispanic Black adults. Understanding whether trends are changing across all tobacco products is increasingly important, given that current tobacco control efforts have reported little success in reducing tobacco use disparities overall. If groups that experience tobacco-related disparities continue to use combustible products while those with higher incomes and education quit or switch to less harmful products, disparities in health outcomes could be exacerbated.

THE NEED FOR TARGETED TOBACCO CONTROL EFFORTS

Reducing disparities has been a public health priority for more than two decades, and some promising frameworks have been identified, such as the social determinants of health approach. However, more work is needed to elucidate effective approaches for reducing tobacco-related disparities at the state and national levels. Examining tobacco use data from states with strong tobacco control programs may help inform efforts to reduce disparities, as these locations may offer an environment more conducive to equitable progress.

In Minnesota, a state with comprehensive and long-term tobacco control programs, data from statewide surveys in 2010, 2014, and 2018 showed no change in disparities by race, education, or income for the use of cigarettes or other tobacco products. These findings are consistent with previous research demonstrating that disparities in cigarette use have remained largely unchanged since 2002 and extend to other tobacco products.

These results highlight two key needs:

1. **Addressing tobacco use beyond cigarettes.** Future tobacco control initiatives and media campaigns should target other tobacco products, such as e-cigarettes and cigars, as patterns of use shift.
2. **Focusing on disproportionately affected communities.** Additional efforts should go beyond policies that have been effective at reducing overall smoking and instead use tailored approaches to target disparately affected communities.

PROMISING POLICY APPROACHES

Some researchers have employed modeling to identify promising approaches to reducing tobacco-related disparities. For example, studies have found that combining restrictions on menthol cigarette sales with buffer zones between retailers could produce a more equitable effect. Literature reviews have also identified that price and tax increases have a consistent, positive influence on socioeconomic inequities for both adults and youth. These models offer important insights but are most valuable when considered alongside real-world policy evaluations.

ADVANCING EQUITY IN TOBACCO CONTROL

As many populations move toward very low levels of cigarette smoking, some have advocated for advancing from conventional tobacco control efforts to more aggressive endgame strategies, such as ending the sale of commercial tobacco. While these approaches have the potential to improve public health broadly and increase equity, some may have unintended consequences. For example, if nicotine reduction policies target only cigarettes and exclude cigars, disparities could be exacerbated among certain groups. Therefore, tobacco control professionals and policymakers must prioritize equity with any proposed strategies and policy initiatives.

Ten years after the passage of the Family Smoking Prevention and Tobacco Control Act, the U.S. Food and Drug Administration (FDA) has yet to exercise its full authority to regulate tobacco products. State and local regulatory efforts will likely be needed for more advanced tobacco policies, such as density policies and those that restrict the sale of flavored tobacco products. A combination of local, state, and federal actions may be the best opportunity for advancing equity.[1]

---

[1] "How Much Progress Have We Made? Trends in Disparities in Tobacco Use," Centers for Disease Control and Prevention (CDC), September 17, 2020. Available online. URL: www.cdc.gov/pcd/issues/2020/20_0090.htm. Accessed September 30, 2024.

Chapter 41 | Promoting Health through Physical Activity for All

Regular physical activity is one of the most important things people can do to improve their health. The recommended amount of physical activity per week varies by age and other factors. Here are the recommendations for different age groups from the *Physical Activity Guidelines for Americans*, 2nd edition. If you are unable to meet the recommendations, be as active as you can.

PHYSICAL ACTIVITY RECOMMENDATIONS FOR CHILDREN

The amount and types of physical activity recommended vary by a child's age.

Children Aged 3–5

- Should be physically active throughout the day for growth and development.
- Adult caregivers should encourage children to be active when they play, such as jumping or riding a tricycle.

Children and Adolescents Aged 6–17

This group needs 60 minutes or more of moderate-to-vigorous intensity physical activity each day, including:

- **Aerobic activity**. Most of the daily 60 minutes or more should include activities such as walking, running, or anything that makes their hearts beat faster. At least three days a week should include vigorous-intensity activities.

- **Muscle-strengthening**. Includes activities such as climbing or doing push-ups, at least three days a week.
- **Bone-strengthening**. Includes activities such as jumping or running, at least three days a week.

An hour of activity a day may sound like a lot, but do not worry! Your children may already be meeting the recommended physical activity levels.

PHYSICAL ACTIVITY RECOMMENDATIONS FOR ADULTS

According to the current *Physical Activity Guidelines for Americans*, adults need 150 minutes of moderate-intensity physical activity a week. This can also be 75 minutes of vigorous-intensity or an equivalent combination of moderate- and vigorous-intensity physical activity. In addition, adults need at least two days of muscle-strengthening activity each week.

We know 150 minutes of physical activity each week sounds like a lot, but you do not have to do it all at once. It could be 30 minutes a day, 5 days a week. You can spread your activity out during the week and break it up into smaller chunks of time.

If you go beyond 150 minutes a week of moderate-intensity activity, or 75 minutes a week of vigorous-intensity activity or an equivalent combination, you will gain even more health benefits.

PHYSICAL ACTIVITY RECOMMENDATIONS FOR OLDER ADULTS

Every week, adults 65 and older need:

- aerobic physical activity that includes:
  - at least 150 minutes at moderate intensity, this could be 30 minutes a day, 5 days a week
  - or 75 minutes at vigorous intensity
  - or an equivalent combination at moderate and vigorous intensity
- at least two days of activities that strengthen muscles
- activities to improve balance

See what counts as aerobic, muscle-strengthening, and balance activities. Also, see how to tell if aerobic physical activity is moderate or vigorous.

If you have trouble meeting these recommendations, be as physically active as your abilities and conditions allow. Remember that some physical activity is better than none at all, and your health benefits will also increase with the more physical activity you do.

Physical activity can prevent or delay many of the health problems that seem to come with age. It also helps your muscles grow stronger so you can keep doing your day-to-day activities without becoming dependent on others.

PHYSICAL ACTIVITY RECOMMENDATIONS FOR PEOPLE WITH CONDITIONS AND DISABILITIES

Regular physical activity provides important health benefits for people with chronic health conditions or disabilities. These people include cancer survivors and those with:

- dementia and other cognitive disorders
- hypertension and stroke
- multiple sclerosis
- osteoarthritis
- Parkinson disease
- spinal cord injury
- type 2 diabetes

Benefits

- Supports daily living activities and independence.
- Improves sleep quality.
- Helps control weight.
- Helps improve mental health by reducing depression and anxiety.
- Lowers the risk for early death, heart disease, type 2 diabetes, and some cancers.
- Decreases pain and improves function in people with osteoarthritis.
- Improves cardiovascular health, muscle fitness, and brain health.

Recommendations

Adults with chronic health conditions or disabilities who are able should: get at least 150 minutes (e.g., 30 minutes, 5 days a week) of moderate-intensity aerobic physical activity per week, and engage in muscle-strengthening activities that include all major muscle groups at least two days per week.

Examples of Physical Activity

- aerobic
  - walking, wheelchair rolling, or biking to places
  - swimming or water aerobics
- muscle-strengthening
  - some yoga postures
  - strengthening exercises using exercise bands, weight machines, or handheld weights

If you have chronic health conditions or disabilities, consult a health-care professional or physical activity specialist about appropriate types and amounts of physical activity.

PHYSICAL ACTIVITY RECOMMENDATIONS FOR PREGNANT AND POSTPARTUM WOMEN

Recommendations

If you are generally healthy, moderate-intensity physical activity is safe for you during pregnancy. It can help reduce your risk of excessive weight gain and gestational diabetes and keep your heart and lungs healthy.

During the postpartum period (first year after delivery), physical activity can decrease symptoms of postpartum depression. When combined with healthy eating, it can also help you with weight loss after delivery.

Get at least 150 minutes (for example, 30 minutes 5 days a week) of moderate-intensity aerobic activity a week during pregnancy and the postpartum period. Remember, some physical activity is better than none, so do what you can.

Benefits

- Reduces the risk of excessive weight gain during pregnancy.
- Reduces the risk of gestational diabetes during pregnancy.
- Reduces symptoms of postpartum depression.

Examples of Physical Activity

- brisk walking
- some forms of yoga
- water aerobics
- bike riding

If you are pregnant, you should be under the care of a doctor who can monitor the progress of the pregnancy. Consult your doctor about whether or how to adjust your physical activity during and after your pregnancy.

Remember that some activity is better than none at all. Incorporating physical activity into your routine can offer numerous health benefits and enhance your overall well-being.[1]

[1] "What You Can Do to Meet Physical Activity Recommendations," Centers for Disease Control and Prevention (CDC), April 16, 2024. Available online. URL: www.cdc.gov/physical-activity-basics/guidelines/index.html. Accessed September 30, 2024.

Chapter 42 | The Importance of Vaccination for Individual and Community Health

From babies to adults, people need vaccines to protect them from potentially dangerous infectious diseases. Without vaccines, children and adults are at risk for serious illness and even death from vaccine-preventable diseases. The U.S. Food and Drug Administration (FDA) has oversight of the safety, effectiveness, and quality of vaccines used in the United States. Vaccines to prevent infectious diseases are administered to millions of babies, children, adolescents, and adults, and it is critical that they meet the FDA's safety and effectiveness standards. Vaccines have prevented countless cases of disease and disability and have saved millions of lives.

THE FDA'S EVALUATION OF VACCINE SAFETY AND EFFECTIVENESS

The FDA's evaluation to determine the safety and effectiveness of vaccines is among the most robust in the world. Vaccine studies are carefully designed to evaluate safety and effectiveness, keeping in mind that millions of people may receive the vaccine. Vaccines do not make you sick with the disease they are preventing. When determining whether to approve or authorize a vaccine for emergency use, the FDA bases its decisions on its analysis of the benefits and risks for the intended population who will receive the vaccine. Vaccines work by mimicking the infectious bacteria or viruses that cause disease. Vaccination stimulates the body's immune system to build up defenses against infectious bacteria or viruses without causing the disease. After vaccination, the immune system is better prepared to respond quickly and forcefully when the body encounters a real disease-causing organism.

VACCINES WORK

Vaccines are effective. Because immunization programs of the 20th and 21st centuries have been so successful, many people today have never seen the various vaccine-preventable diseases that were once common, including polio, diphtheria, rubella (German measles), and chickenpox.

VACCINES SAVE LIVES

Infectious diseases that once killed or harmed many infants, children, and adults could reemerge if people are not vaccinated. The germs (viruses and bacteria) that cause vaccine-preventable diseases still exist and can harm people who are not vaccinated.

VACCINATION HELPS PROTECT COMMUNITIES

If too many individuals choose not to vaccinate themselves or their children, some diseases that are now rare or nonexistent in the United States may resurface. For example, measles is one of the most contagious respiratory diseases in the world and has the potential to be life-threatening for some people. Outbreaks in the United States continue to occur because measles is common in many parts of the world, unvaccinated travelers with measles are bringing the disease into the United States from other countries, and measles can spread in communities in the United States where groups of people are unvaccinated.

MOST SIDE EFFECTS FROM VACCINES ARE MILD

Vaccines are medical products. Like any medicine, vaccines can cause side effects. However, most side effects are minor and short-lived, such as a low-grade fever or pain and redness at the injection site. Vaccines are safe, and severe side effects are rare. The risk of being harmed by vaccines is much smaller than the risk of serious illness from the diseases they prevent. Let your health-care professional know about any questions or concerns you have about vaccines.

There are real dangers to the health of individuals who are unvaccinated. Some people are surprised to learn that children can be harmed by or even die from measles, influenza, and other diseases that can be prevented by vaccines.[1]

[1] "Vaccine Facts: Why You and Your Family Need Vaccines," U.S. Food and Drug Administration (FDA), August 29, 2023. Available online. URL: www.fda.gov/media/171671/download. Accessed September 30, 2024.

Chapter 43 | Strengthening Vaccine Confidence

Child vaccination coverage remains high nationally, and most parents are confident in vaccine safety and effectiveness. However, the spread of myths and misinformation has put some communities at risk. When misleading information circulates, vaccination coverage can fall and increase the risk of outbreaks of vaccine-preventable diseases.

CDC APPROACH

Vaccinate with Confidence is the Centers for Disease Control and Prevention's (CDC) strategic framework for strengthening vaccine confidence and preventing outbreaks of vaccine-preventable diseases in the United States. It combines the CDC's existing work with new investments, partnerships, and activities to protect communities at risk and strengthen public trust in vaccines' life-saving protection.

Vaccinate with Confidence will strengthen public trust in vaccines by advancing three key priorities:

Protect Communities

Vaccination rates remain strong nationally, but pockets of under-vaccination persist in some locations, putting communities at risk for outbreaks. The CDC will support states, cities, and counties to find these communities and take steps to protect them.

Empower Families

Trust in vaccines is not built through a top-down approach but through millions of conversations among parents, doctors, nurses, pharmacists, and community members. The CDC will expand resources for health-care professionals to support effective vaccine conversations.

Stop Myths

To stop misinformation from eroding public trust in vaccines, the CDC will work with local partners and trusted messengers to improve confidence in vaccines among at-risk groups; establish partnerships to contain the spread of misinformation; and reach critical stakeholders to provide clear information about vaccination and the critical role it plays in protecting the public.

CDC VACCINATION STRATEGY

Protect Communities

The CDC is supporting partners to find and protect communities at risk.

NEW INVESTMENTS AND PARTNERSHIPS

- Leverage the CDC's Immunization and Vaccines for Children cooperative agreement to support efforts to find and respond to pockets of low vaccine coverage.
- Use immunization information system data to pinpoint areas of low vaccination coverage.
- Build immunization program capacity and leadership to effectively respond to outbreaks.

Empower Families

The CDC is working with key partners to strengthen parent-provider conversations about vaccines.

NEW INVESTMENTS AND PARTNERSHIPS

- Start vaccine conversations earlier, with parents of very young infants and pregnant women.
- Reduce hesitancy and improve vaccine access at the nation's community health centers.
- Develop a provider toolkit to address parents' vaccine questions during outbreaks.

Stop Myths

The CDC is engaging local messengers and partners to contain the spread of misinformation and ensure key stakeholders have critical information about vaccines.

NEW INVESTMENTS AND PARTNERSHIPS

- Work with social media companies to promote trustworthy vaccine information.
- Provide accurate, accessible information on vaccines to state policymakers.
- Engage state and local health officials to advance effective local responses to misinformation.

Priorities for 2020 and Beyond

The CDC will prioritize the activities below to ensure that every community is protected:

- Leverage diverse data sources to find and protect communities at risk.
- Expand resources for working with local communities.
- Build and foster a culture of immunization in health-care practices.
- Continually improve communication strategies.
- Further invest in and collaborate with vital partners.

COVID-19 STATE OF VACCINE CONFIDENCE

The CDC regularly creates reports about the status of coronavirus 2019 (COVID-19) vaccine confidence in the United States, emphasizing major themes that influence vaccine confidence and uptake. The reports include analyses of multiple quantitative and qualitative data sources, ranging from social listening and web metrics to immunization survey data and CDC-INFO inquiries.[1]

---

[1] "Vaccinate with Confidence," Centers for Disease Control and Prevention (CDC), October 30, 2019. Available online. URL: www.cdc.gov/vaccines/partners/vaccinate-with-confidence.html. Accessed September 30, 2024.

Chapter 44 | Improving Care for Individuals with Multiple Chronic Conditions

CHRONIC ILLNESS AND MULTIPLE CHRONIC CONDITIONS

Chronic illness, particularly among individuals with multiple chronic conditions (MCC), accounts for the majority of health-care expenditures and is usually associated with poor quality of care—because the care of these individuals is often fragmented, incomplete, inefficient, and ineffective. Because people with MCC suffer suboptimal health care and incur rising health-care expenses, enhanced attention on this population is critical to improve health-care quality and reduce costs.

HHS MULTIPLE CHRONIC CONDITIONS INITIATIVE

In December 2010, the U.S. Department of Health and Human Services (HHS), with input from key stakeholder organizations, released an action-oriented strategic framework that outlines strategies for maximizing care of and improving health and quality of life for individuals with MCC.

On March 27, 2012, an expert panel was convened at HHS to identify and prioritize strategies outlined in the MCC Strategic Framework requiring more intensive activity. The panel felt that shared learning of efforts to appropriately identify and stratify high-risk patient populations, particularly patients with MCC, for more focused care interventions would be a positive step toward addressing a gap of activity in the MCC Strategic Framework.

IDENTIFICATION AND MANAGEMENT OF HIGH-RISK INDIVIDUALS

Disease and care management models have evolved to manage costs while improving the care of individuals with chronic conditions. These models use various means to identify and stratify patients for targeted interventions, including:

- predictive modeling software
- emergency department (ED) utilization
- specific clinical conditions
- clinician referrals
- risk assessments

Claims-based predictive modeling tools are data-driven decision-support tools that attempt to estimate or predict individuals' future health-care costs and health-care utilization based on multiple factors, including prior health service utilization and chronic illness burden. Other, more accessible methods for identifying individuals who are at high risk for poor outcomes or increased health-care utilization include self-administered and clinician-administered health assessments or disease counts.

Often, programs or models combine strategies to identify cohorts of patients and tailor interventions to patients' needs. For example, they combine information on ED use, hospitalizations, costs, and clinical conditions to identify appropriate patients. Patients may be further stratified to more or less intensive care management based on their diagnostic and utilization profile.

Questions remain, however, about which data elements improve predictive accuracy and how these may vary for different subpopulations (e.g., Medicaid vs. Medicare vs. general populations). For instance, studies have shown that methods that simply rely on identifying current high utilizers (e.g., individuals with one or more ED admissions in the previous year) are not good predictors of future utilization. Others have shown that the inclusion of variables such as functional status, illness severity, behavioral health status, and social determinants of health are important for accurately identifying individuals with the greatest risk. However, there are challenges with obtaining and integrating this type of information into current tools.

Other questions of interest relate to identifying patients (e.g., frail elderly, individuals with co-occurring behavioral health conditions, or physical disabilities) who could best benefit from higher versus lower touch interventions. A number of recent care management interventions and models have attempted to prioritize the level of outreach and intensity of care based on an individual's risk level. Some models with demonstrated effectiveness target interventions on individuals who are in periods of transition (e.g., discharge from an acute care hospital) or who change their current risk level. Which approaches are most effective for specific subgroups of individuals with MCC remain unclear. Additionally, how can risk identification be conducted effectively in real time to potentially facilitate the implementation of targeted interventions where and when they are needed?

Addressing the challenges in identifying and managing high-risk individuals with multiple chronic conditions is essential for improving health-care quality and reducing costs. By exploring effective strategies for risk prediction and tailored interventions, health-care providers can better serve this population. Continued research and shared learning are necessary to determine the most effective approaches for different subgroups and to implement real-time risk identification.[1]

[1] "Identifying and Stratifying Individuals with Multiple Chronic Conditions for Care Management," U.S. Department of Health and Human Services (HHS), August 15, 2012. Available online. URL: www.hhs.gov/sites/default/files/ash/initiatives/mcc/implementation/aug2012-summary.pdf. Accessed September 25, 2024.

Chapter 45 | Telehealth Interventions for Managing Chronic Diseases

OVERVIEW

The Community Preventive Services Task Force (CPSTF) recommends several telehealth interventions for reducing chronic disease risk factors in patients and managing chronic diseases or conditions. These conditions include:

- cardiovascular disease
- high blood pressure (HBP)
- diabetes
- HIV (human immunodeficiency virus) infection
- end-stage renal disease
- asthma
- obesity

The CPSTF found that the use of telehealth interventions can improve:

- medication adherence, such as outpatient follow-up and self-management goals
- clinical outcomes, such as blood pressure control
- dietary outcomes, such as eating more fruits and vegetables and reducing sodium (salt) intake

Components of telehealth that have been shown to be effective include:

- text messaging, such as tailored patient education and medication and appointment reminders
- web-based content and applications, such as goal-setting and reminder functions on mobile phones
- interactive content, such as patients sending health data to their health-care provider

HIGHLIGHTS

Telehealth involves health-care delivery and education over a distance using electronic and telecommunication technologies. Telehealth aims to be an integral method of providing health-care services to the public.

Currently, telehealth can be delivered in several different ways. For example:

- **Live (synchronous) videoconferencing**. This is typically a two-way audiovisual link between health-care providers or between a patient and a provider. For example, stroke specialists at different hospitals can communicate about transferring a patient with a stroke from one hospital to another for more specialized care.
- **Store-and-forward (asynchronous) videoconferencing**. This is an exchange of recorded patient health information between providers or between a patient and a provider. For example, community pharmacists can send recommendations about medicines to a patient's provider through secure email or a patient portal.
- **Remote patient monitoring (RPM)**. This is the use of electronic devices to record a patient's health data for a provider to receive and evaluate at a later time. For example, a patient can use RPM to measure their blood pressure regularly and send this information to their provider.
- **mHealth**. This refers to health-related applications and programs used on mobile phones and other

smart devices. For example, mHealth can include text messages or phone applications that help patients manage their blood pressure and cholesterol levels.
- **Audio only**. This refers to the use of a landline or mobile phone to connect a patient to a provider. For example, a provider and patient can talk directly about how the patient can manage a chronic disease, condition, or risk factor.

Definitions and policies about what can be covered and reimbursed by public and private insurers also differ. Because definitions of telehealth vary, not every delivery method may be considered telehealth in every jurisdiction. Issues related to patient privacy and confidentiality must also be considered for each method.[1]

[1] "Telehealth Interventions to Improve Chronic Disease," Centers for Disease Control and Prevention (CDC), May 15, 2024. Available online. URL: www.cdc.gov/cardiovascular-resources/php/data-research/telehealth.html. Accessed September 25, 2024.

Chapter 46 | **Advancing Health Equity through CDC's Strategic Initiatives**

The Centers for Disease Control and Prevention (CDC) works to ensure health equity is embedded in an all-of-public health approach to overcoming persistent health disparities and health inequities across a range of population groups that disproportionately experience poor health outcomes.

PARTNERSHIPS TO ADVANCE HEALTH EQUITY

- In 2023, the CDC launched a health equity partnership network in collaboration with the Association of State and Territorial Health Officials (ASTHO) and the National Association of State Offices of Minority Health (NASOMH). This network, the "Power of Partnerships," mobilizes health equity partners within local Offices of Minority Health, Offices of Women's Health/Maternal and Child Health, community-based organizations, and nongovernmental organizations, and assists communities across the country with meeting local health needs, especially during emergency situations.
  - **Impact**. Through this network, multidisciplinary teams engage to share information on implementing evidence-based practices and policies that advance the health and well-being of people who have experienced

historical discrimination and oppression across jurisdictions.

- In 2023, the CDC launched a series of health equity partnership webinars (www.cdc.gov/health-equity/events/partnerwebinar.html) to bring together an intersectional collective of health equity organizations that focus on a range of populations, including racial and ethnic minorities, people with disabilities, LGBTQ+ people, and more.
  - **Impact.** Public health and health-care partners learn about and apply promising health equity strategies in their communities through these informative webinars. Since 2023, over 2,500 partners have joined for sessions on the respiratory virus response season and health equity communications—the series will continue throughout 2024.

BUILDING HEALTH EQUITY INTO CDC SCIENCE

- In 2023, the CDC published an article on CDC's Health Equity Science Principles, which introduces health equity science as a conceptual framework to advance health equity and describes six principles to guide the development, implementation, dissemination, and use of effective health equity science.
  - **Impact.** The Health Equity Science Principles establish an equity-focused scientific framework to guide researchers inside and outside the CDC looking to address equity through public health science. Leaders are applying these equity principles in public health surveillance, research, and evaluation.
- In 2023, the CDC collaborated with multiple community partners through its "Communities in Context" program in the Greater Detroit, Michigan, area to pilot a public health monitoring framework and track structural drivers of inequities at the local level to identify areas for improving community health.
  - **Impact.** Communities in Context improves public health decision-making by identifying shared priorities

for action and creating publicly available and user-friendly resources that communities can use to support informed action.

- In 2023, the CDC launched the Health Equity Science Manuscript Development Program, an in-service program that supports CDC scientists who show promise in advancing health equity through scientific projects. The part-time, six–to–eight-month program focused on health equity science involves mentoring and training in the development of impactful health equity scientific publications. Participants produce at least one peer-reviewed scientific manuscript focused on a priority health equity science issue and a related scientific presentation.
  - **Impact**. The Health Equity Science Manuscript Development Program is helping to develop a cadre of scientists focused on establishing the evidence base for programs and policies that advance health equity.

ADVANCING COMMUNICATION IN HEALTH EQUITY

- In 2022, the CDC conducted message testing to learn more about what various audiences think, understand, and feel about the concept of health equity and ways to create effective messages for specific audiences. The message testing informed three communication principles (www.cdc.gov/health-equity/what-is/communicating.html) that help to switch the conversation from naming and quantifying health disparities to addressing health equity.
  - **Impact**. Communicating using a health equity frame means focusing on creating a broader understanding of the social, structural, and systemic factors that may influence health outcomes.
- In 2022, to further advance communication about health equity, the CDC developed a series of videos (www.cdc.gov/health-equity/what-is/video.html) to explain health equity and related concepts, including social determinants of health, racism and health, and intersectionality.

Together, this series of videos provides a more complete picture of what health equity is, why it is important to advance health equity as part of a complete public health approach, and provides a tool for public health practitioners, academics, and decision makers to use when explaining these complicated topics.

- **Impact.** The videos improve partners' understanding of health equity; since being uploaded in 2023, they have been shared widely (nearly 100,000 views).

HEALTH EQUITY EMERGENCY RESPONSE CADRE

- During the coronavirus 2019 (COVID-19) response, the CDC introduced a new position, the Chief Health Equity Officer (CHEO), into its Incident Management Structure to address COVID-19-associated health disparities in morbidity and mortality caused by systemic and structural inequities. Starting in 2023, the CDC Office of Readiness and Response ensures that agency-led responses include a Chief Health Equity Officer (CHEO) position or unit in order to address health disparities and inequities.
    - **Impact.** The CHEO role has helped to ensure that health disparities data were examined and reported on to inform the development of culturally relevant recommendations for populations more heavily affected by COVID-19. Additional health equity roles have been identified as part of a response cadre and will be integrated into each CDC task force and unit to ensure standard implementation of the health equity strategy for future emergency responses.

CDC DIVERSITY, EQUITY, INCLUSION, ACCESSIBILITY (DEIA) STRATEGIC PLAN

- In 2022, the CDC launched its Antiracism and Health Sprint Team to strengthen institutional subject matter expertise and equity infrastructure as part of the CDC's DEIA Strategic Action Plan.

- **Impact**. The Sprint Team works to ensure that the CDC operationalizes best practices for intersectional racial equity.

- In response to Executive Order 14035 on Diversity, Equity, Inclusion, and Accessibility in the Federal Workplace and the release of the Government-wide Strategic Plan to Advance Diversity, Equity, Inclusion, and Accessibility in the Federal Workforce in 2021, the CDC developed an agency-specific DEIA Strategic Plan to emphasize its commitment to developing a workforce and workplace that represents equity principles and furthers efforts to achieve the public health mission.
    - **Impact**. This plan led to the establishment of one competency, "Diversity, Equity, Inclusion & Accessibility Management," that has been identified as critical and has been integrated into the CDC's Career+ pilot. Additionally, it informed the development and implementation of an employee DEIA training curriculum, convening of an annual DEIA–Equal Employment Opportunity forum for all employees, and increased participation in DEIA councils, CDC organizations and associations, workgroups, and special emphasis programs. The agency now annually recognizes the people, workgroups, and organizations facilitating DEIA via the DEIAB and EEO Workplace Equity Innovation Award. A diverse hiring panel tool is being implemented to standardize and automate the way in which diverse résumé review and interview panels are formed. The goal is to sustain a culture where the workforce has an enhanced social and cultural understanding of the communities served while also infusing diversity, equity, inclusion, and accessibility in all aspects of the agency's work.[1]

[1] "Health Equity," Centers for Disease Control and Prevention (CDC), July 18, 2024. Available online. URL: www.cdc.gov/health-equity/core/health-equity-fact-sheet.html. Accessed September 25, 2024.

Chapter 47 | Advancing Health Equity through HHS's Strategic Initiatives

IMPROVING HEALTH OUTCOMES

The U.S. Department of Health and Human Services (HHS) is committed to addressing health disparities and advancing health equity by expanding access to care, improving health-care quality, and supporting health-care providers who serve populations who are at increased risk for poor health outcomes.

Quality Affordable Maternal Health Care

The United States has the highest maternal mortality rate among developed nations, and Native Hawaiian and other Pacific Islanders, Black, American Indian, and Alaska Native individuals have the highest rates of pregnancy-related deaths. HHS is committed to improving maternal health and advancing health equity.

- Medicaid and the Children's Health Insurance Program (CHIP) finance more than 4 in 10 births in the United States and are an important source of maternal health care. The HHS has encouraged states to take up a new option to extend postpartum coverage under Medicaid and CHIP from 60 days to 12 months. Thus far, 45 states plus Washington, D.C., and the U.S. Virgin Islands have expanded postpartum coverage.
- In September 2023, the Health Resources and Services Administration (HRSA) announced nearly $90 million in awards to increase access to care in maternity care

deserts, address maternal depression, and grow the maternal health workforce.
- In 2023, the HHS reached a milestone of more than 1,900 birthing facilities participating in the Alliance for Innovation on Maternal Health, a program under which hospitals and other facilities adopt proven strategies to increase safe births and reduce negative birth outcomes.
- The HHS has invested in and made HHS's new maternity care quality data easily accessible through the Care Compare "Birthing-Friendly" designation, a consumer-friendly icon noting that a hospital or health system has demonstrated a commitment to improving maternity care quality.
- In 2023, the HHS reached a milestone of supporting 36 Perinatal Quality Collaboratives (PQCs). PQCs are state or multistate networks of multidisciplinary teams working to improve population-level maternal and infant health care and outcomes statewide. PQCs advance evidence-based clinical practices and processes using quality improvement principles and convene and collaborate with diverse representatives (clinical teams, experts, partners, patients, families) to rapidly improve perinatal health care and outcomes statewide and reduce disparities in health care and outcomes between subpopulations within a state.

Improved Health Outcomes for People with HIV

The United States is making progress toward eliminating HIV (human immunodeficiency virus) transmission, but these efforts must be accelerated.

- Through the HRSA Ryan White HIV/AIDS Program (RWHAP), nearly 9 out of 10 people with HIV who receive RWHAP medical services reached viral suppression in 2022. This means that they cannot transmit HIV to their partners and these people can live longer, healthier lives. The percentage of Black/African-American clients, Hispanic/Latino clients, and youth and young adult clients aged 13–24 who received care through the RWHAP and reached viral suppression all far exceeded overall national viral suppression rates.

- Due in part to the efforts of multiple HHS agencies to expand pre-exposure prophylaxis (PrEP) awareness, availability, and provider capacity, preliminary data indicate that in 2022, 36 percent of the 1.2 million people who could benefit from PrEP were prescribed it, compared to 23 percent in 2019, the year that the Ending the HIV Epidemic in the U.S. (EHE) Initiative was announced.
- The Centers for Disease Control and Prevention's (CDC's) EHE-funded programs have provided more than 44,000 PrEP prescriptions and connected with over 260 Syringe Services Programs (SSPs), 60 percent of which provide mobile services.
- In 2020 and 2021, HRSA's RWHAP served nearly 38,000 clients new to care or re-engaged in care in support of the EHE. In the first two years of EHE, more than 20 percent of people in EHE jurisdictions who were undiagnosed or not previously in care were served by HRSA-funded EHE providers.
- The Substance Abuse and Mental Health Services Administration (SAMHSA) funded three Minority HIV/AIDS Fund: Integrated Behavioral Health and HIV Care for Unsheltered Populations Pilot Project grants in fiscal year 2023 for a total of $1,997,536. The program provides comprehensive health care and addresses disparities facing medically underserved people experiencing unsheltered homelessness through portable clinical care delivered outside that is focused on the integration of behavioral health and HIV treatment and prevention services.

Addressing and Improving Outcomes for Sickle Cell Disease

Sickle cell disease (SCD) is the most common inherited blood disorder in the United States, affecting more than 100,000 Americans and disproportionately affecting Black and Hispanic/Latino Americans.

- From data collection and research to the approval of new therapies, the HHS is answering the call and supporting programs critical for helping people with SCD live healthier lives. Ongoing efforts include expanding the Sickle Cell Data Collection program; releasing a Sickle Cell Disease Action Plan; continuing research on treatment including through the Cure Sickle Cell Initiative; supporting programs that span across the SCD system of care, such as newborn screening, diagnosis, and access to treatments; and considering testing approaches to improve access to innovative treatments and reduce program expenditures starting with SCD under the Cell and Gene Therapy Access model recently announced by the CMS Innovation Center.

ADVANCING DATA EQUITY

Health equity data can help care teams identify and address health disparities, leading to improved health outcomes at the individual and population levels. Data can streamline social care referrals and improve care delivery, person-centered decision-making, research, population health improvement, and public health. The privacy interests of American Indian and Alaska Native populations should be respected when working with tribal communities.

Standardizing Social Determinants of Health and Sexual Orientation and Gender Identity Data

The Office of the National Coordinator for Health Information Technology (ONC) U.S. Core Data for Interoperability (USCDI) is a standardized set of health data elements for nationwide, interoperable health information exchange. Starting in 2026, much-certified health information technology (IT) products will need to support new data elements that promote health equity, including sexual orientation and gender identity (SOGI) data and social determinants of health assessment data, such as assessments of housing and food insecurity risk.

Collecting Information That Strengthens Our Understanding of the Drivers of Inequities in Maternal Mortality

The CDC's Enhancing Reviews and Surveillance to Eliminate Maternal Mortality (ERASE MM) program supports standardized data collection across Maternal Mortality Review Committees (MMRCs) active in states and territories to understand the circumstances of all pregnancy-related deaths and strategies for prevention. In addition to adding fields to specifically capture discrimination and racism in the Maternal Mortality Review Information Application (MMRIA), the CDC worked with the HHS Office of Minority Health and other partners to develop and implement a web portal for MMRCs to view "Community Vital Signs" dashboards that provide increased community details and context (e.g., obstetricians or nurse midwives per capita, unmet need for drug treatment, poverty rate, community levels of education, violent crime rates) to MMRCs during their review of each death.

Transparent Use of Equity-Related Health Information

Since ONC launched the Health IT Certification Program in 2010, almost all U.S. hospitals and close to 80 percent of office-based physicians use certified electronic health records. ONC recently established first-of-its-kind transparency requirements for artificial intelligence and other predictive algorithms that are part of certified health IT to the decision support intervention certification criterion. The HHS's leading-edge regulatory approach promotes the safe development and use of artificial intelligence, machine learning, and predictive clinical decision support by promoting health equity and fairness and identifying issues of bias.[1]

---

[1] "Advancing Health Equity across HHS," U.S. Department of Health and Human Services (HHS), May 21, 2024. Available online. URL: www.hhs.gov/equity/fact-sheet-advancing-health-equity-across-hhs/index.html. Accessed September 25, 2024.

Part 7 | Additional Help and Information

Chapter 48 | Glossary of Demographic and Health-Related Terms

acquired immunodeficiency syndrome (AIDS): A condition where the immune system cannot defend the body against infections. It is caused by the human immunodeficiency virus (HIV), which is spread through contact with infected blood or body fluids. High-risk activities include unprotected sexual intercourse and intravenous drug use. There is no cure, but research on vaccines is ongoing.

anxiety: Feelings of fear, restlessness, or unease, often as a response to stress. Symptoms may include sweating, tension, and rapid heartbeat.

asthma: A chronic condition causing inflammation and constriction of the airways, leading to difficulty breathing, wheezing, and coughing.

bacteria: Microscopic organisms, some of which cause infections or diseases in humans and animals.

bone marrow: Soft tissue found inside bones that produces blood cells, including those that fight infections.

cancer: A group of diseases where abnormal cells grow uncontrollably, potentially spreading to other parts of the body.

caregiver: A person who provides care for an elderly individual or someone with a disability at home.

cholesterol: A substance found in animal-based foods and the bloodstream that is necessary for cellular function, but excessive levels can increase the risk of heart disease.

This glossary contains terms excerpted from documents produced by several sources deemed reliable.

chronic pain: Persistent or recurring pain that lasts for extended periods, ranging from mild to severe.

clinical trial: A research study that tests new medical interventions in people to assess their safety and effectiveness.

counseling: A professional process to help people manage mental, emotional, or personal issues.

cultural competency: The ability of health-care providers to deliver services that meet the social, cultural, and linguistic needs of patients.

culture: The collective beliefs, values, behaviors, and customs of a group, which are passed down through generations and continually evolve.

cystic fibrosis (CF): A genetic disease that causes thick mucus buildup, affecting organs such as the lungs and pancreas.

deoxyribonucleic acid (DNA): The molecule that carries genetic information in all living organisms.

depression: A mental health condition marked by persistent feelings of sadness, hopelessness, and a lack of interest in daily activities.

diabetes: A chronic condition where the body is unable to regulate blood sugar levels due to insufficient insulin production or use.

disparities in health care: Differences in health-care access, quality, and outcomes among different population groups.

environmental justice: The fair treatment and meaningful involvement of all people in environmental policy-making, regardless of race or income.

ethnicity: A person's cultural, linguistic, or racial heritage.

exercise: Planned, structured physical activity that is performed to improve or maintain physical fitness.

health equity: The effort to eliminate health-care disparities and provide equal access to health-care services for all populations.

heart disease: A range of conditions that affect the heart, including coronary artery disease, which can lead to heart attacks.

hemochromatosis: A condition where excess iron builds up in the body, potentially damaging organs.

hepatitis B: A viral infection that affects the liver, transmitted through blood or other bodily fluids.

hepatitis C: A viral infection of the liver, spread mainly through blood contact.

human immunodeficiency virus (HIV): The virus that attacks the immune system and causes AIDS.

hypertension: Also known as "high blood pressure" (HBP), it is when the force of blood against artery walls is too high, potentially causing health issues.

infection: The invasion and multiplication of germs, such as bacteria or viruses, in the body.

life expectancy: The average number of years an individual is expected to live based on demographic factors.

Medicaid: A joint federal and state program that provides health-care coverage to individuals with limited income and resources.

mental health services: Services aimed at supporting individuals with emotional or mental health issues, provided by professionals in health-care settings.

migration: Movement of individuals who leave their region of residence to live in another region.

mortality rate: The number of deaths in a population over a given time.

nursing home: A residential facility for people who need assistance with daily living but do not require hospital care.

nutrition: The study of how food and its components affect health and wellness.

obesity: Having an excessive amount of body fat, often defined as a "body mass index" (BMI) of 30 or higher.

osteoporosis: A condition where bones become weak and brittle due to low bone mass.

outpatient: A patient who receives medical treatment without being admitted to the hospital.

physical activity: Any movement that uses skeletal muscles and requires energy expenditure.

population health: The health outcomes of a group of individuals, including the distribution of these outcomes.

preterm birth: Birth that occurs before the 37th week of pregnancy.

quality of life: The general well-being of an individual, encompassing physical, mental, and social aspects.

race: A social construct used to group people into a hierarchical human-grouping system. This system generates racial classifications to identify, distinguish, and marginalize certain groups across nations, regions, and the world. It divides human populations into groups often based on physical appearance, social factors, and cultural backgrounds.

screening test: A preliminary test used to identify individuals who may have or be at risk for a particular disease or condition.

social determinants of health (SDOH): The conditions in which people live, work, and grow that influence health outcomes.

social service: A community resource that helps people access services such as health care, transportation, and home care.

socioeconomic status: A measure of an individual's or group's access to collectively desired resources, including economic, social, and cultural capital. It is a fundamental construct in the social and health sciences, influencing various aspects of life, such as health outcomes, education, and quality of life.

stroke: A medical emergency where the blood supply to the brain is interrupted, leading to loss of function or death.

structural racism: Policies and practices embedded in institutions that create unequal access to opportunities and resources based on race.

tuberculosis (TB): A bacterial infection primarily affecting the lungs, spread through airborne particles.

vaccination: The injection of a weakened or dead pathogen to prevent future infection.

Chapter 49 | Directory of Organizations and Resources for Health Equity and Support

GOVERNMENT ORGANIZATIONS

Agency for Healthcare Research and Quality (AHRQ)
5600 Fishers Ln.
7th Fl.
Rockville, MD 20847
Phone: 301-427-1104
Website: www.ahrq.gov

Centers for Disease Control and Prevention (CDC)
1600 Clifton Rd., N.E.
Atlanta, GA 30329
Toll-Free: 800-CDC-INFO
(800-232-4636)
Phone: 770-488-1725
Toll-Free TTY: 888-232-6348
Website: www.cdc.gov
Email: hrcs@cdc.gov

Federal Trade Commission (FTC)
600 Pennsylvania Ave., N.W.
Washington, DC 20580
Toll-Free: 877-FTC-HELP
(877-382-4357)
Phone: 202-326-2222
Website: www.ftc.gov

Health Resources and Services Administration (HRSA)
5600 Fishers Ln.
Rockville, MD 20857
Toll-Free: 877-464-4772
Website: www.hrsa.gov

HealthCare.gov
Toll-Free: 800-318-2596
Toll-Free TTY: 855-889-4325
Website: www.healthcare.gov

Resources in this chapter were compiled from several sources deemed reliable; all contact information was verified and updated in November 2024.

HIV.gov
1101 Wootton Pkwy.
Rockville, MD 20852
Toll-Free: 800-HIV-0440
(800-448-0440)
Website: www.hiv.gov
Email: contact@hiv.gov

MedlinePlus
8600 Rockville Pike
Bethesda, MD 20894
Toll-Free: 888-FIND-NLM
(888-346-3656)
Phone: 301-594-5983
Website: www.medlineplus.gov

National Cancer Institute (NCI)
9609 Medical Center Dr.
Bethesda, MD 20892-9760
Toll-Free: 800-4-CANCER
(800-422-6237)
Website: www.cancer.gov
Email: NCIinfo@nih.gov

National Endowment for the Humanities (NEH)
400 Seventh St., S.W.
Washington, DC 20506
Phone: 202-606-8400
Toll-Free TTY: 800-877-8399
Website: www.neh.gov
Email: questions@neh.gov

National Heart, Lung, and Blood Institute (NHLBI)
P.O. Box 30105
Bethesda, MD 20824
Toll-Free: 877-NHL-BI4U
(877-645-2448)
Website: www.nhlbi.nih.gov
Email: nhlbiinfo@nhlbi.nih.gov

National Human Genome Research Institute (NHGRI)
Bldg. 31, Rm. 4B09
31 Center Dr., MSC 2152
9000 Rockville Pike
Bethesda, MD 20892-2152
Phone: 301-402-0911
Fax: 301-402-2218
Website: www.genome.gov
Email: nhgripressoffice@mail.nih.gov

National Institute of Diabetes and Digestive and Kidney Diseases (NIDDK)
9000 Rockville Pike
Bethesda, MD 20892
Toll-Free: 800-860-8747
Website: www.niddk.nih.gov
Email: healthinfo@niddk.nih.gov

National Institute of General Medical Sciences (NIGMS)
45 Center Dr.
MSC 6200
Bethesda, MD 20892-6200
Phone: 301-496-7301
Website: www.nigms.nih.gov

National Institute of Mental Health (NIMH)
6001 Executive Blvd.
MSC 9663
Bethesda, MD 20892-9663
Toll-Free: 866-615-6464
Website: www.nimh.nih.gov
Email: nimhinfo@nih.gov

National Institute on Alcohol Abuse and Alcoholism (NIAAA)
Toll-Free: 888-MY-NIAAA
(888-696-4222)
Phone: 301-443-3860
Website: www.niaaa.nih.gov
Email: AskNIAAA@nih.gov

National Institute on Minority Health and Health Disparities (NIMHD)
6707 Democracy Blvd., Ste. 800
Bethesda, MD 20892-5465
Phone: 301-402-1366
Fax: 301-480-4049
Website: www.nimhd.nih.gov
Email: NIMHDinfo@NIMHD.NIH.gov

National Park Service (NPS)
1849 C St., N.W.
Washington, DC 20240
Phone: 202-208-6843
Website: www.nps.gov

Office of Minority Health (OMH)
1101 Wootton Pkwy, Ste. 600
Tower Oaks Bldg.
Rockville, MD 20852
Phone: 833-762-4900
TDD: 301-251-1432
Fax: 240-453-8812
Website: https://minorityhealth.hhs.gov

Substance Abuse and Mental Health Services Administration (SAMHSA)
5600 Fishers Ln.
Rockville, MD 20857
Toll-Free: 877-SAMHSA-7
(877-726-4727)
Toll-Free TTY: 800-487-4889
Website: www.samhsa.gov
Email: SAMHSAInfo@samhsa.hhs.gov

U.S. Bureau of Labor Statistics (BLS)
2 Massachusetts Ave., N.E., Ste. 2135
Washington, DC 20212-0001
Phone: 202-691-6500
Fax: 202-691-6444
Website: www.bls.gov

U.S. Census Bureau
4600 Silver Hill Rd.
Suitland, MD 20746
Toll-Free: 800-923-8282
Phone: 301-763-INFO
(301-763-4636)
Toll-Free TDD/TTY:
800-877-8339
Website: www.census.gov

U.S. Department of Health and Human Services (HHS)
200 Independence Ave., S.W.
Hubert H. Humphrey Bldg.
Washington, DC 20201
Toll-Free: 877-696-6775
Website: www.hhs.gov

U.S. Food and Drug Administration (FDA)
10903 New Hampshire Ave.
Silver Spring, MD 20993
Toll-Free: 888-INFO-FDA
(888-463-6332)
Phone: 301-796-8240
Website: www.fda.gov

PRIVATE ORGANIZATIONS

American Lung Association (ALA)
55 W. Wacker Dr., Ste. 1150
Chicago, IL 60601
Toll-Free: 800-LUNGUSA (800-586-4872)
Website: www.lung.org
Email: info@lung.org

American Society of Hispanic Economists (ASHE)
Website: https://asheweb.org

Asian and Pacific Islander American Health Forum (APIAHF)
1444 I St., N.W., Ste. 700
Washington, DC 20005
Phone: 202-466-7772
Website: www.apiahf.org
Email: info@apiahf.org

ASPIRA Association
1220 L St., N.W., Ste. 701
Washington, DC 20005
Website: https://aspira.org
Email: info@aspira.org

Association of Naval Services Officers (ANSO)
Website: www.ansomil.org

The Center for Advancing Health (CFAH)
Website: www.cfah.org

The Center for Asian Pacific American Women (CAPAW)
1160 Battery St., E., Ste. 100
San Francisco, CA 94111
Website: https://capaw.org
Email: info@capaw.org

Center for Health, Environment & Justice (CHEJ)
P.O. Box 6806
Falls Church, VA 22040-6806
Phone: 703-237-2249
Website: https://chej.org
Email: info@chej.org

Community Catalyst
Two Liberty Square
11th Fl.
Boston, MA 02109
Phone: 617-338-6035
Website: https://communitycatalyst.org

Congressional Hunger Center
200 Massachusetts Ave., N.W.
7th Fl.
Washington, DC 20001
Phone: 202-547-7022
Fax: 202-547-7575
Website: https://hungercenter.org

Grantmakers in Health (GIH)
1100 Connecticut Ave., N.W., Ste. 1100
Washington, DC 20036
Phone: 202-452-8331
Website: www.gih.org

Institute for the Advancement of Multicultural & Minority Medicine (IAMMM)
1218 16 St., N.W.
Washington, DC 20036
Phone: 202-667-6155
Fax: 202-667-6156
Website: https://iammm.org
Email: info@iammm.org

Joint Center for Political and Economic Studies
633 Pennsylvania Ave., N.W.
Washington, DC 20004
Phone: 202-789-3500
Website: https://jointcenter.org
Email: info@jointcenter.org

National Black Nurses Association (NBNA)
8630 Fenton St., Ste. 910
Silver Spring, MD 20910
Phone: 301-589-3200
Fax: 301-589-3223
Website: https://nbna.org
Email: info@nbna.org

National CARES Mentoring Movement
5 Penn Plaza
23rd Fl.
New York, NY 10001
Phone: 212-629-0737
Website: www.caresmentoring.org
Email: info@caresmentoring.org

National Center for Children in Poverty (NCCP)
475 Riverside Dr., Ste. 1400
New York, NY 10115
Website: www.nccp.org

National Center for Healthy Housing (NCHH)
10320 Little Patuxent Pkwy.
Ste. 200
Columbia, MD, 21044
Phone: 410-992-0712
Website: https://nchh.org

National Council of Asian Pacific Americans (NCAPA)
1612 K St., N.W., Ste. 600
Washington, DC 20006
Website: www.ncapaonline.org
Email: info@ncapaonline.org

National Health Law Program
1444 I St., N.W., Ste. 1105
Washington, DC 20005
Phone: 202-289-7661
Website: https://healthlaw.org

National Medical Association (NMA)
8403 Colesville Rd.
Ste. 820
Silver Spring, MD 20910
Phone: 202-347-1895
Fax: 301-495-0359
Website: www.nmanet.org

National Minority Quality Forum (NMQF)
1201 15th St., N.W., Ste. 340
Washington, DC 20005
Phone: 202-223-7560
Website: https://nmqf.org
Email: infodesk@nmqf.org

Population Reference Bureau
1111 19th St., N.W., Ste. 400
Washington, DC 20036
Phone: 800-877-9881
Website: www.prb.org
Email: communications@prb.org

Society for Public Health Education (SOPHE)
10 G St., N.E., Ste. 605
Washington, DC 20002
Phone: 202-408-9804
Fax: 202-408-9815
Website: www.sophe.org
Email: info@sophe.org

Society for the Analysis of African American Public Health Issues (SAAPHI)
P.O. Box 7712
York, PA 17404
Website: www.saaphi.org
Email: saaphipr@gmail.com

UnidosUS
1126 16th St., N.W., Ste. 600
Washington, DC 20036
Phone: 202-785-1670
Website: https://unidosus.org
Email: info@unidosus.org

INDEX

INDEX

Page numbers followed by "n" refer to citation information; by "t" indicate tables; and by "f" indicate figures.

A

B

C

D

F

G

H

I

J

K

L

M

N

P

T

W